PANSS
培训教材

上海市精神卫生中心　药物临床试验培训中心　编写

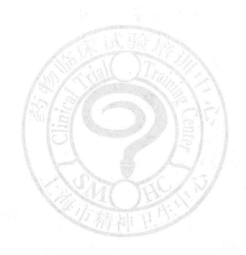

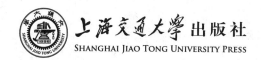

上海交通大学 出版社
SHANGHAI JIAO TONG UNIVERSITY PRESS

内容提要

PANSS(阳性和阴性症状量表)是当前精神科最常使用的量表之一。在 20 世纪 90 年代即通过翻译后在中国开始广泛应用。但该量表的正确使用对于评分员要求较高,通常需要具有一定工作经验的精神科医生接受规范培训并通过一致性测试后,方可使用。本书的出版旨在促进和规范 PANSS 的教学和培训,以便提高所有涉及使用 PANSS 的临床研究的质量。本书不仅适用于精神科临床研究的培训和操作,也可作为医学工作者的学术参考。

图书在版编目(CIP)数据

PANSS 培训教材/上海市精神卫生中心药物临床试验
培训中心编写. —上海:上海交通大学出版社,2017
ISBN 978 - 7 - 313 - 16960 - 0

Ⅰ.①P… Ⅱ.①上… Ⅲ.①精神病学-教材
Ⅳ.①R749

中国版本图书馆 CIP 数据核字(2017)第 108058 号

PANSS 培训教材

编　　写:	上海市精神卫生中心药物临床试验培训中心			
出版发行:	上海交通大学出版社	地　　址:	上海市番禺路 951 号	
邮政编码:	200030	电　　话:	021 - 64071208	
出 版 人:	郑益慧			
印　　制:	常熟市文化印刷有限公司	经　　销:	全国新华书店	
开　　本:	787mm×1092mm 1/16	印　　张:	7	
字　　数:	151 千字			
版　　次:	2017 年 6 月第 1 版	印　　次:	2017 年 6 月第 1 次印刷	
书　　号:	ISBN 978 - 7 - 313 - 16960 - 0/R			
定　　价:	38.00 元			

版权所有　侵权必究
告读者:如发现本书有印装质量问题请与印刷厂质量科联系
联系电话:0512 - 52219025

前　言

众所周知,精神医学的研究对象是人类的高级精神活动,因此精神卫生领域的临床诊断和疗效评价不可避免地带有主观色彩。要想尽可能地克服这种主观偏倚,规范使用量表(Rating Scales)是一种切实可行的手段,也只有这样才能使量表成为真正有价值的评价工具,最终保障临床研究数据的真实和可靠。

PANSS 全称 Positive and Negative Syndrome Scale(阳性和阴性症状量表)是针对精神分裂症临床研究最常使用的量表工具。1987 年由 Stanley R. Kay、Lewis A. Opler 和 Abraham Fiszbein 研制,2000 年进行修订,2002 年增加了知情者调查问卷(IQ-PANSS)。

1996 年,PANSS 最早由西安杨森公司引入中国,之后在中国的精神药物临床试验中开始应用,并逐渐扩展至各种精神卫生临床研究。但该量表的正确使用对于评分员要求较高,通常需要具有一定工作经验的精神科医生接受规范培训并通过一致性测试后,方可使用。因此出版本书旨在促进和规范 PANSS 的教学和培训,以便提高所有涉及使用 PANSS 的临床研究的质量。本书不仅适用于精神科临床研究的培训和操作,也可作为医学工作者的学术参考。

该项工作是李华芳教授领衔的课题组承接国家十一五和十二五"重大新药创制"科技重大专项——精神药物新药临床评价研究技术平台(2008—2015)的一个重要建设内容。沈一峰、李妍、余一旻、于文娟、王志阳参加了本书的编写工作。

上海市精神卫生中心药物临床试验培训中心编写组

2017.4

目　录

PASS

第一章

PANSS 简介

PANSS 于 1987 年由 Stanley R. Kay、Lewis A. Opler 和 Abraham Fiszbein 研制。其来源是 1962 年 Overall. J. E 和 Gorham. D. R 研制的 BPRS（the Brief Psychiatric Rating Scale，简明精神症状评定量表），以及 1975 年 Singh. M. M 和 Kay. S. R 研制的 PRS（Psychopathology Rating Schedule，精神病理学评定日程表）。

PANSS 之前的相关量表（例如目前仍在用的 BPRS）中，阳性症状和阴性症状项目数不平衡，也没有指标反映患者症状中是阳性还是阴性占优势，研制 PANSS 的初衷即在于解决该问题；同时 PANSS 也形成了每个条目的操作用评分标准，有助于精确评估症状严重程度；还建立了配套的标准化检查（SCI-PANSS），有利于规范收集信息进行完整评估。

PANSS 一经推出，迅速成为精神分裂症研究中的主要评价工具。至 2000 年，PANSS 进行修订。2002 年，又增加了知情者调查问卷（IQ-PANSS），进一步完善信息的收集。因此，完整的 PANSS 工具包括 3 个部分，PANSS、SCI-PANSS 和 IQ-PANSS。本教材会分章节介绍。

PANSS 总计包括 33 条目，分四大类：阳性量表（P）7 项，阴性量表（N）7 项，一般精神病理量表（G）16 项，以及攻击危险性的补充项目 3 项。最后 3 项较少使用，临床研究中通常使用前 30 项。具体条目名称、内容和操作性分级标准，详见第二章。需要注意的是，PANSS 每个条目的评分等级是 7 级：1～7，即使该条目评分内容完全没有，也是评 1 分，而不是评 0 分。因此，PANSS 总分的最小值为 30 分，出现低于该数值的情况，均需强调规范培训。

PANSS 评分信息的来源，各个条目有所不同。仅根据知情者信息的 2 项：N4，G16；需要结合现场检查和知情者信息的 12 项：P1，P3，P4，P5，P6，P7，N2，G5，G6，G7，G8，G14；只根据现场检查信息的 16 项：P2，N1，N3，N5，N6，N7，G1，G2，G3，G4，G9，G10，G11，G12，G13，G15。

SCI-PANSS（Structured Clinical Interview for PANSS）即 PANSS 的定式化临床检查，通过结构式访谈的设计，指导评分员如何询问和探查症状，以保证收集信息的完整和可信。SCI-PANSS 专门用于收集评定所需的临床资料，通常要求结合临床实际，通过自如的互相交流获得相关信息，因此只有经过专门临床训练的精神科医生才能胜任。一般需要 30～40 分钟。访谈用模板（文字稿）详见第三章。

IQ-PANSS（Informant Questionnaire for PANSS）即 PANSS 知情者调查问卷，是通过主要知情者，包括家人、护士和其他人员（同学、老师、同事、邻居等），了解评分相关信息。使用 IQ-PANSS 既能提高信度，节约时间；又能参考和补充信息，对于准确评分有益（详见第四章）。需要指出，PANSS 是一个典型的他评量表，无论评分相关信息来源如何，通常均由评分员对相关信息进行综合判断后进行评定。因此，知情者信息≠评分（除外 N4 和 G16）。

PANSS 作为评价指标用于临床研究时，除通常使用的 PANSS 总分外，还可以根据研究目的使用一些因子分。例如 PANSS-EC（兴奋因子），包括 P4、G4、P7、G8、G14，常被用于评估精神分裂症患者的兴奋激越。

Marder 教授根据自己的研究，又把 PANSS 的 30 个条目重新分为 5 个维度：

维度 1	阴性症状	Negative Symptoms	N1、N2、N3、N4、N6、G7、G16
维度 2	阳性症状	Positive Symptoms	P1、P3、P5、P6、N7、G1、G9、G12
维度 3	思维紊乱	Disorganized Thought	P2、N5、G5、G10、G11、G13、G15
维度 4	无法控制的敌对/兴奋	Uncontrolled Hostility/Excitement	P4、P7、G8、G14
维度 5	焦虑/抑郁	Anxiety/Depression	G2、G3、G4、G6

PANSS 引入中国以后，被广泛用于精神分裂症的临床研究中。查询中国知网期刊全文库，使用关键词"精神分裂症"和"PANSS"，可以查见文献超过 5 000 多篇，其中学术期刊 4 764，博士论文 41，硕士论文 190，会议论文 343。表明 PANSS 在中国已被普遍使用。

因为在培训和临床研究应用中均发现，一些具体使用问题的源头来自翻译，因此本教材尽可能地提供了英文原文，便于使用者对中文量表（翻译）有疑问时可参照原文进行理解。一些国际研究中，甚至会明确以英文量表为准，中文仅供参考。

PANSS

Fill in the appropriate circle for each item, refer to the Rating Manual for item definitions, description of anchoring points and scoring procedure.

一 Positive Scale (P)

P1. Delusions

Beliefs which are unfounded, unrealistic, and idiosyncratic.

Basis for rating: thought content expressed in the interview and its influence on social relations and behavior as reported by primary care workers or family.

	Rating	Criteria
1	Absent	Definition does not apply
2	Minimal	Questionable pathology; may be at the upper extreme of normal limits
3	Mild	Presence of one or two delusions, which are vague, uncrystallized, and not tenaciously held. Delusions do not interfere with thinking, social relations, or behavior
4	Moderate	Presence of either a kaleidoscopic array of poorly formed, unstable delusions or a few well-formed delusions that occasionally interfere with thinking, social relations, or behavior
5	Moderate Severe	Presence of numerous well-formed delusions that are tenaciously held and occasionally interfere with thinking, social relations, or behavior
6	Severe	Presence of a stable set of delusions which are crystallized, possibly systematized, tenaciously held, and clearly interfere with thinking, social relations, and behavior
7	Extreme	Presence of a stable set of delusions which are either highly systematized or very numerous, and which dominate major facets of the patient's life. This frequently results in inappropriate and irresponsible action, which may even jeopardize the safety of the patient or others

P2. Conceptual disorganization

Disorganized process of thinking characterized by disruption of goal-directed sequencing, e. g., circumstantiality, tangentiality, loose associations, non-sequiturs, gross illogicality, or thought block.

Basis for rating: cognitive-verbal processes observed during the course of interview.

第二章

PANSS

根据评估手册中每一项条目的定义、评分要点和信息来源,对下列每一项进行恰当的评定。

一 阳性量表

P1. 妄想

妄想是指无事实根据、与现实不符、特异的信念。

评分依据: 会谈中患者思维的自然表达,及由基层保健工作者或家属提供的其思维对社会交往和行为造成的影响。

	分级	标　　准
1	无	定义不适用于该患者
2	很轻	症状可疑,但可能是正常范围的上限
3	轻度	存在一个或两个模糊的、不具体的、并非顽固坚持的妄想,妄想不妨碍思考、社交关系或行为
4	中度	存在一个多变的、未完全成形的、不稳定的妄想组合,或几个完全成形的妄想,偶尔妨碍思考、社交关系或行为
5	偏重	存在许多完全成形的且顽固坚持的妄想,偶尔妨碍思考、社交关系或行为
6	重度	存在一整套稳定的、具体的妄想,可能系统化,顽固坚持,且明显妨碍思考、社交关系和行为
7	极重度	存在一整套高度系统化或数量众多的稳定的妄想,并支配患者生活的主要方面,以至常引起不恰当的和不负责任的行为,甚至可能因此危及患者或他人的安全

◆ P1 评定妄想性思维的存在、严重性和干扰程度,不评定妄想性思维可能伴有的异常行为或偏执狂。

P2. 概念紊乱

思维过程紊乱,其特征为思维的目的性、连贯性破坏,如赘述、离题、联想散漫、不连贯、显著的不合逻辑,或思维阻隔。

评分依据: 会谈中观察患者的认知-言语表达过程。

	Rating	Criteria
1	Absent	Definition does not apply
2	Minimal	Questionable pathology; may be at the upper extreme of normal limits
3	Mild	Thinking is circumstantial, tangential, or paralogical. There is some difficulty in directing thoughts toward a goal, and some loosening of associations may be evidenced under pressure
4	Moderate	Able to focus thoughts when communications are brief and structured, but becomes loose or irrelevant when dealing with more complex communications or when under minimal pressure
5	Moderate Severe	Generally has difficulty in organizing thoughts, as evidenced by frequent irrelevancies, disconnectedness, or loosening of associations even when not under pressure
6	Severe	Thinking is seriously derailed and internally inconsistent, resulting in gross irrelevancies and disruption of thought processes, which occur almost constantly
7	Extreme	Thoughts are disrupted to the point where the patient is incoherent. There is marked loosening of associations, which results in total failure of communication, e. g., "word salad" or mutism

P3. Hallucinatory behavior

Verbal report or behavior indicating perceptions which are not generated by external stimuli. These may occur in the auditory, visual, olfactory, or somatic realms.

Basis for rating: verbal report and physical manifestations during the course of interview as well as reports of behavior by primary care workers or family.

	Rating	Criteria
1	Absent	Definition does not apply
2	Minimal	Questionable pathology; may be at the upper extreme of normal limits
3	Mild	One or two clearly formed but infrequent hallucinations, or else a number of vague abnormal perceptions, which do not result in distortions of thinking or behavior
4	Moderate	Hallucinations occur frequently but not continuously, and the patient's thinking and behavior are affected only to a minor extent
5	Moderate Severe	Hallucinations are frequent, may involve more than one sensory modality, and tend to distort thinking and/or disrupt behavior. Patient may have delusional interpretation of these experiences and respond to them emotionally and, on occasion, verbally as well
6	Severe	Hallucinations are present almost continuously, causing major disruption of thinking and behavior. Patient treats these as real perceptions, and functioning is impeded by frequent emotional and verbal responses to them
7	Extreme	Patient is almost totally preoccupied with hallucinations, which virtually dominate thinking and behavior. Hallucinations are provided a rigid delusional interpretation and provoke verbal and behavioral responses, including obedience to command hallucinations

	分级	标　　准
1	无	定义不适用于该患者
2	很轻	症状可疑,但可能是正常范围的上限
3	轻度	思维显得不直接、离题或逻辑障碍,思维的目的性有些障碍,在压力下显得有些联想散漫
4	中度	当交谈短暂和有序时尚可集中思维,当交谈较复杂或有轻微压力时就变得散漫或离题
5	偏重	普遍存在构思困难,在无压力时也经常显得离题、不连贯或联想散漫
6	重度	思维严重出轨及自相矛盾,导致明显的离题和思维中断,几乎是持续出现
7	极重度	思维中断至支离破碎的程度,明显的联想散漫,导致完全无法交谈,如"语词杂拌"或缄默

◆ 妄想性思维可能思维还组织得很好,问你自己:"这一思维内容合乎情理吗?"
◆ "压力"指在追问下或对问题加以澄清时。

P3. 幻觉性行为

语言表达或行为表明存在非外部刺激引起的知觉,这些知觉可以听觉、视觉、嗅觉或躯体感觉的形式出现。

评分依据：会谈中患者的语言表达和躯体表现,也可由基层保健工作者或家属提供的患者情况。

	分级	标　　准
1	无	定义不适用于该患者
2	很轻	症状可疑,但可能是正常范围的上限
3	轻度	一种或两种清晰但不经常出现的幻觉,或若干模糊异常的知觉,尚未引起思维或行为的失常
4	中度	幻觉频繁但并不持续出现,患者的思维和行为仅受到轻微影响
5	偏重	幻觉频繁出现,可能涉及一种以上感觉系统,导致思维失常和(或)妨碍行为;患者可能对这些体验给予妄想性的解释,并出现情绪反应,偶尔出现语言反应
6	重度	幻觉几乎持续存在,以致严重损害思维和行为,患者对这些幻觉信以为真,频繁的情绪和语言反应导致功能障碍
7	极重度	患者几乎沉浸在幻觉中,幻觉几乎支配患者的思维和行为,幻觉被赋予固定的妄想性解释,并引起言语和行为上的反应,包括对命令性幻听的服从

◆ 评定依据为幻觉的存在和频度及对患者行为的影响(干扰)。

P4. Excitement

Hyperactivity as reflected in accelerated motor behavior，heightened responsivity to stimuli，hypervigilance，or excessive mood lability.

Basis for rating：behavioral manifestations during the course of interview as well as reports of behavior by primary care workers or family.

	Rating	Criteria
1	Absent	Definition does not apply
2	Minimal	Questionable pathology; may be at the upper extreme of normal limits
3	Mild	Tends to be slightly agitated，hypervigilant，or mildly overaroused throughout the interview，but without distinct episodes of excitement or marked mood lability. Speech may be slightly pressured
4	Moderate	Agitation or overarousal is clearly evident throughout the interview，affecting speech and general mobility，or episodic outbursts occur sporadically
5	Moderate Severe	Significant hyperactivity or frequent outbursts of motor activity are observed，making it difficult for the patient to sit still for longer than several minutes at any given time
6	Severe	Marked excitement dominates the interview，delimits attention，and to some extent affects personal functions such as eating and sleeping
7	Extreme	Marked excitement seriously interferes in eating and sleeping and makes interpersonal interactions virtually impossible. Acceleration of speech and motor activity may result in incoherence and exhaustion

P5. Grandiosity

Exaggerated self-opinion and unrealistic convictions of superiority，including delusions of extraordinary abilities，wealth，knowledge，fame，power，and moral righteousness.

Basis for rating：thought content expressed in the interview and its influence on behavior as reported by primary care workers or family.

	Rating	Criteria
1	Absent	Definition does not apply
2	Minimal	Questionable pathology; may be at the upper extreme of normal limits
3	Mild	Some expansiveness or boastfulness is evident，but without clear-cut grandiose delusions
4	Moderate	Feels distinctly and unrealistically superior to others. Some poorly formed delusions about special status or abilities may be present but are not acted upon
5	Moderate Severe	Clear-cut delusions concerning remarkable abilities，status，or power are expressed and influence attitude but not behavior
6	Severe	Clear-cut delusions of remarkable superiority involving more than one parameter（wealth，knowledge，fame，etc.）are expressed，notably influence interactions，and may be acted upon
7	Extreme	Thinking，interactions，and behavior are dominated by multiple delusions of amazing ability，wealth，knowledge，fame，power，and/or moral stature，which may take on a bizarre quality

P4. 兴奋

活动过度,表现在动作行为加速,患者对刺激的反应增强,高度警觉或过度的情绪不稳。

评分依据:根据会谈过程中患者动作行为的表现,也可由基层保健工作者或家属提供的患者状况。

	评分	标 准
1	无	定义不适用于该患者
2	很轻	症状可疑,但可能是正常范围的上限
3	轻度	会谈中患者呈轻度的激越、警觉增高,或轻度的激动,但没有明显兴奋或情绪不稳的发作,讲话有轻微的紧迫感
4	中度	会谈中患者出现明显的激越或激动,影响语言和一般动作或偶有短暂的爆发
5	偏重	观察到患者明显的活动过度或频繁的动作行为爆发,以致患者在任何时候都难以保持坐姿超过数分钟
6	重度	会谈中患者明显兴奋,注意力受限,在某种程度上影响个人功能,诸如饮食和睡眠
7	极重度	患者有明显的兴奋严重妨碍饮食和睡眠,并使得人际交往实际上变得不可能。言语和动作行为的加速可能导致语无伦次和精疲力竭

◆ 指行为方面的表现:活动增多、易激惹,不包括言语和思维的兴奋。

P5. 夸大

夸张己见及不切实际的优势观念,包括一些妄想,如非凡的能力、财富、知识、名望、权力和道德止义。

评分依据:会谈中患者思维的自然表达,及由基层保健工作者或家属提供的这些想法对患者行为的影响。

	评分	标 准
1	无	定义不适用于该患者
2	很轻	症状可疑,但可能是正常范围的上限
3	轻度	显出有些自大或自夸,但没有明确的夸大妄想
4	中度	明显地和不切实际地感到自己比他人优越,有一些尚未成形的关于特殊地位或能力的妄想,但并未照此行动
5	偏重	患者表现出明显的关于非凡能力、地位或权利的妄想,影响患者的态度,但不影响行为
6	重度	患者表现出涉及到一个以上的项目(财富、知识、名望等),有明确的显著优势妄想,明显影响人际交往,并可能付诸行动
7	极重度	患者的思维、人际交往和行为受多重妄想的支配,这些妄想包括惊人的能力、财富、知识、名望、权力和(或)道德高度,可能具有古怪的性质

P6. Suspiciousness/persecution

Unrealistic or exaggerated ideas of persecution, as reflected in guardedness, a distrustful attitude, suspicious hypervigilance, or frank delusions that others mean one harm.

Basis for rating: thought content expressed in the interview and its influence on behavior as reported by primary care workers or family.

	Rating	Criteria
1	Absent	Definition does not apply
2	Minimal	Questionable pathology; may be at the upper extreme of normal limits
3	Mild	Presents a guarded or even openly distrustful attitude, but thoughts, interactions, and behavior are minimally affected
4	Moderate	Distrustfulness is clearly evident and intrudes on the interview and/or behavior, but there is no evidence of persecutory delusions. Alternatively, there may be indication of loosely formed persecutory delusions, but these do not seem to affect the patient's attitude or interpersonal relations
5	Moderate Severe	Patient shows marked distrustfulness, leading to major disruption of interpersonal relations, or else there are clear-cut persecutory delusions that have limited impact on interpersonal relations and behavior
6	Severe	Clear-cut pervasive delusions of persecution which may be systematized and significantly interfere in interpersonal relations
7	Extreme	A network of systematized persecutory delusions dominates the patient's thinking, social relations, and behavior

P7. Hostility.

Verbal and nonverbal expressions of anger and resentment, including sarcasm, passive-aggressive behavior, verbal abuse, and assaultiveness.

Basis for rating: interpersonal behavior observed during the interview and reports by primary care workers or family.

	Rating	Criteria
1	Absent	Definition does not apply
2	Minimal	Questionable pathology; may be at the upper extreme of normal limits
3	Mild	Indirect or restrained communication of anger, such as sarcasm, disrespect, hostile expressions, and occasional irritability
4	Moderate	Presents an overtly hostile attitude, showing frequent irritability and direct expression of anger or resentment
5	Moderate Severe	Patient is highly irritable and occasionally verbally abusive or threatening
6	Severe	Uncooperativeness and verbal abuse or threats notably influence the interview and seriously impact upon social relations. Patient may be violent and destructive but is not physically assaultive toward others
7	Extreme	Marked anger results in extreme uncooperativeness, precluding other interactions, or in episode(s) of physical assault toward others

P6. 猜疑或被害感

不切实际或夸大的被害观念,患者表现在防卫、不信任态度、多疑的高度戒备,或是认为他人对其有伤害,显示患者有非常明显的妄想。

评分依据:会谈中患者思维的自然表达,及由基层保健工作者或家属提供的对其行为的影响。

	评分	标　　准
1	无	定义不适用于该患者
2	很轻	症状可疑,但可能是正常范围的上限
3	轻度	患者表现出防卫或甚至公开的不信任态度,但思维、交往和行为只受到最小限度的影响
4	中度	患者明确地显示出不信任感,并妨碍会谈和(或)行为,但没有被害妄想的证据;或者,可能存在结构松散的被害妄想,但这些似乎不影响患者的态度或人际关系
5	偏重	患者表现出明显的不信任感,以致人际关系造成严重破坏,或者还存在明确的被害妄想,对人际关系和行为造成有限的影响
6	重度	患者有明确的泛化的被害妄想,可能是系统化的,且显著地妨碍人际关系
7	极重度	一整套系统性被害妄想支配患者的思维、社交关系和行为

◆ 须区分因情感疏离或淡漠性退缩所致的防卫。

P7. 敌对性

愤怒和怨恨的言语和非言语表达,包括讥讽、被动攻击行为、辱骂和袭击。

评分依据:会谈中观察患者的人际行为,及由基层保健工作者或家属提供的患者情况。

	评分	标　　准
1	无	定义不适用于该患者
2	很轻	症状可疑,但可能是正常范围的上限
3	轻度	间接地或经过克制地表示愤怒,如讥讽,不尊敬,表达敌意及偶尔易激惹
4	中度	存在明显敌对态度,经常表现易激惹及直接表达愤怒或怨恨
5	偏重	患者高度易激惹,而且偶尔有辱骂或言语威胁
6	重度	不合作和辱骂或言语威胁显著地影响会谈,且严重影响社交关系,患者可能具有暴力和破坏性,但没有对他人进行人身攻击
7	极重度	明显的愤怒造成极度不合作,拒绝与他人交往或对他人进行人身攻击

◆ 指被害妄想引起的敌意,敌对的对象可以是任何人。

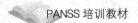

二 —— Negative Scale (N)

N1. Blunted affect

Diminished emotional responsiveness as characterized by a reduction in facial expression, modulation of feelings, and communicative gestures.

Basis for rating: observation of physical manifestations of affective tone and emotional responsiveness during the course of interview.

	Rating	Criteria
1	Absent	Definition does not apply
2	Minimal	Questionable pathology; may be at the upper extreme of normal limits
3	Mild	Changes in facial expression and communicative gestures seem to be stilted, forced, artificial, or lacking in modulation
4	Moderate	Reduced range of facial expression and few expressive gestures result in a dull appearance
5	Moderate Severe	Affect is generally "flat," with only occasional changes in facial expression and a paucity of communicative gestures
6	Severe	Marked flatness and deficiency of emotions exhibited most of the time. There may be unmodulated extreme affective discharges, such as excitement, rage, or inappropriate uncontrolled laughter
7	Extreme	Changes in facial expression and evidence of communicative gestures are virtually absent. Patient seems constantly to show a barren or "wooden" expression

N2. Emotional withdrawal

Lack of interest in, involvement with, and affective commitment to life's events.

Basis for rating: reports of functioning from primary care workers or family and observation of interpersonal behavior during the course of interview.

	Rating	Criteria
1	Absent	Definition does not apply
2	Minimal	Questionable pathology; may be at the upper extreme of normal limits
3	Mild	Usually lacks initiative and occasionally may show deficient interest in surrounding events
4	Moderate	Patient is generally distanced emotionally from the milieu and its challenges but, with encouragement, can be engaged
5	Moderate Severe	Patient is clearly detached emotionally from persons and events in the milieu, resisting all efforts at engagement. Patient appears distant, docile, and purposeless but can be involved in communication at least briefly and tends to personal needs, sometimes with assistance
6	Severe	Marked deficiency of interest and emotional commitment results in limited conversation with others and frequent neglect of personal functions, for which the patient requires supervision
7	Extreme	Patient is almost totally withdrawn, uncommunicative, and neglectful of personal needs as a result of profound lack of interest and emotional commitment

二　阴性量表

N1. 情感迟钝

情感反应减弱，以面部表情、感觉调节及体态语言的减少为特征。

评分依据： 会谈中观察患者情感基调和对情绪反应所产生的躯体表现。

	评分	标　准
1	无	定义不适用于该患者
2	很轻	症状可疑，但可能是正常范围的上限
3	轻度	面部表情和体态语言似乎显得呆板、勉强、做作，或缺少变化
4	中度	面部表情和体态语言的减少使患者看上去迟钝
5	偏重	情感总体上显得"平淡"，面部表情仅偶尔有所变化，缺乏体态语言
6	重度	大部分时间表现明显的情感平淡和缺乏情绪表达，可能存在无法调控的极端情感发泄，如兴奋、愤怒或不恰当的无法控制的发笑
7	极重度	完全缺乏面部的表情和体态语言，患者似乎持续地显示出木讷的表情或毫无表情

◆ 指情感的非言语表达，不仅观察面部表情，而且还有姿势动作，应除外药物引起的 EPS 症状。
◆ 6 分包括缺乏情感调节及情绪反应平淡。

N2. 情绪退缩

对生活事件缺乏兴趣、参与和情感投入。

评分依据： 由基层保健工作者或家属提供，及会谈中观察到的患者所表现的人际行为。

	评分	标　准
1	无	定义不适用于该患者
2	很轻	症状可疑，但可能是正常范围的上限
3	轻度	患者常缺乏主动性，偶尔显得对周围事件缺乏兴趣
4	中度	患者总体上对周围环境及环境变化有情感隔阂，但给予鼓励仍可参与
5	偏重	患者对周围的人和事有明显的情感疏远，抵制所有的参与努力，患者显得疏远、温顺和漫无目的，但至少可进行短暂的交流，倾向于个人需求，有时需要帮助
6	重度	明显的缺乏兴趣和情感投入，导致患者与他人交谈有限，并且经常忽略个人功能，因此患者需要监督
7	极重度	兴趣和情感投入的极度缺乏导致患者几乎完全退缩，无法交谈，并忽略个人需求

◆ 评估跟生活事件有关的情感退缩应包括对个人功能的忽视。
◆ 须区别 N2 和 N4（社交退缩），后者更多地聚焦于由知情者报告的因淡漠、缺乏精力和意志力而致社交兴趣和主动性的下降。

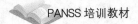

N3. Poor rapport

Lack of interpersonal empathy, openness in conversation, and sense of closeness, interest, or involvement with the interviewer. This is evidenced by interpersonal distancing and reduced verbal and nonverbal communication.

Basis for rating: interpersonal behavior during the course of interview.

	Rating	Criteria
1	Absent	Definition does not apply
2	Minimal	Questionable pathology; may be at the upper extreme of normal limits
3	Mild	Conversation is characterized by a stilted, strained or artificial tone. It may lack emotional depth or tend to remain on an impersonal, intellectual plane
4	Moderate	Patient typically is aloof, with interpersonal distance quite evident. Patient may answer questions mechanically, act bored, or express disinterest
5	Moderate Severe	Disinvolvement is obvious and clearly impedes the productivity of the interview. Patient may tend to avoid eye or face contact
6	Severe	Patient is highly indifferent, with marked interpersonal distance. Answers are perfunctory, and there is little nonverbal evidence of involvement. Eye and face contact are frequently avoided
7	Extreme	Patient is totally uninvolved with the interviewer. Patient appears to be completely indifferent and consistently avoids verbal and nonverbal interactions during the interview

N4. Passive/apathetic social withdrawal

Diminished interest and initiative in social interactions due to passivity, apathy, anergy, or avolition. This leads to reduced interpersonal involvements and neglect of activities of daily living.

Basis for rating: reports on social behavior from primary care workers or family.

	Rating	Criteria
1	Absent	Definition does not apply
2	Minimal	Questionable pathology; may be at the upper extreme of normal limits
3	Mild	Shows occasional interest in social activities but poor initiative. Usually engages with others only when approached first by them
4	Moderate	Passively goes along with most social activities but in a disinterested or mechanical way. Tends to recede into the background
5	Moderate Severe	Passively participates in only a minority of activities and shows virtually no interest or initiative. Generally spends little time with others
6	Severe	Tends to be apathetic and isolated, participating very rarely in social activities and occasionally neglecting personal needs. Has very few spontaneous social contacts
7	Extreme	Profoundly apathetic, socially isolated, and personally neglectful

N3. 情感交流障碍

缺乏人际交往中的感情投入、交谈时的坦率及亲密感、兴趣或与会谈者的互动,患者表现在人际关系疏远及语言和非语言交流的减少。

评分依据: 会谈中的患者所表现的人际行为能力。

	评分	标　　准
1	无	定义不适用于该患者
2	很轻	症状可疑,但可能是正常范围的上限
3	轻度	交谈以呆板、紧张或音调不自然为特征,患者可能缺乏情绪深度或倾向于停留在非个人的、理智性的水平
4	中度	患者显出典型的冷淡,人际关系疏远相当明显,患者可能机械地回答问题,表现为不耐烦或表示无兴趣
5	偏重	明显的不投入并妨碍到会谈的词汇表达量,患者可能避开眼神的接触或面部表情的交流
6	重度	患者显得高度冷漠,有明显的人际疏远,回答问题敷衍,很少有投入会谈的非言语迹象,常常避开眼神的接触和面部表情的交流
7	极重度	患者完全不投入会谈,显得完全冷漠,会谈中始终回避言语和非言语交流

◆ 指在检查交谈时,无法实现正常的情感交流,在患者与检查者之间存在一道无形的隔膜。

N4. 被动性或淡漠性社交退缩

因被动、淡漠、缺乏精力或意志力使社会交往的兴趣和主动性下降,这导致人际交往的减少及对日常活动的忽视。

评分依据: 由基层保健工作者或家属提供的患者的社会行为情况。

	评分	标　　准
1	无	定义不适用于该患者
2	很轻	症状可疑,但可能是正常范围的上限
3	轻度	患者显示对社交活动偶有兴趣,但主动性较差,通常只有在他人先主动表示时才会参与
4	中度	被动地参与大部分的社交活动,但以无兴趣或机械的方式出现,倾向于退缩到不显眼的地方
5	偏重	仅被动参与少数活动,且实际上显得毫无兴趣或主动性,通常只花很少时间与他人相处
6	重度	趋于淡漠和孤立,极少参与社交活动,偶尔忽视个人需求,很少有自发的社交接触
7	极重度	极度的淡漠,与世隔绝,且忽视个人需求

◆ 为阴性症状病征的核心特征。

◆ 须区别 N4 和 G16(主动回避社交),后者是评估与恐惧、敌意或不信任有关的社交参与的减少。

N5. Difficulty in abstract thinking

Impairment in the use of the abstract-symbolic mode of thinking, as evidenced by diffculty in classification, forming generalizations, and proceeding beyond concrete or egocentric thinking in problem-solving tasks.

Basis for rating: responses to questions on similarities and proverb interpretation, and use of concrete vs. abstract mode during the course of the interview.

	Rating	Criteria
1	Absent	Definition does not apply
2	Minimal	Questionable pathology; may be at the upper extreme of normal limits
3	Mild	Tends to give literal or personalized interpretations to the more difficult proverbs and may have some problems with concepts that are fairly abstract or remotely related
4	Moderate	Often utilizes a concrete mode. Has difficulty with most proverbs and some categories. Tends to be distracted by functional aspects and salient features
5	Moderate Severe	Deals primarily in a concrete mode, exhibiting difficulty with most proverbs and many categories
6	Severe	Unable to grasp the abstract meaning of any proverbs or figurative expressions and can formlulate classifications for only the most simple of similarities. Thinking is either vacuous or locked into functional aspects, salient features, and idiosyncratic interpretations
7	Extreme	Can use only concrete modes of thinking. Shows no comprehension of proverbs, common metaphors or similes, and simple categories. Even salient and functional attributes do not serve as a basis for classification. This rating may apply to those who cannot interact even minimally with the examiner due to marked cognitive impairment

N6. Lack of spontaneity and flow of conversation

Reduction in the normal flow of communication associated with apathy, avolition, defensiveness, or cognitive deficit. This is manifested by diminished fluidity and productivity of the verbal-interactional process.

Basis for rating: cognitive-verbal processes observed during the course of interview.

	Rating	Criteria
1	Absent	Definition does not apply
2	Minimal	Questionable pathology; may be at the upper extreme of normal limits
3	Mild	Conversation shows little initiative. Patient's answers tend to be brief and unembellished, requiring direct and leading questions by the interviewer
4	Moderate	Conversation lacks free flow and appears uneven or halting. Leading questions are frequently needed to elicit adequate responses and proceed with conversation
5	Moderate Severe	Patient shows a marked lack of spontaneity and openness, replying to the interviewer's questions with only one or two brief sentences
6	Severe	Patient's responses are limited mainly to a few words or short phrases intended to avoid or curtail commununication. (E. g., "I don't know," "I'm not at liberty to say.") Conversation is seriously impaired as a result, and the interview is highly unproductive
7	Extreme	Verbal output is restricted to, at most, an occasional utterance, making conversation impossible

N5. 抽象思维困难

运用抽象-象征性思维模式受损,表现在分类、概括及解决问题时超越具体或自我中心的思维过程出现困难。

评分依据:会谈中患者回答相似性问题和解释谚语类问题的能力,及运用具体对抽象模式的情况。

	评分	标　　准
1	无	定义不适用于该患者
2	很轻	症状可疑,但可能是正常范围的上限
3	轻度	对较难懂的谚语倾向于按照字面或给予个人化的解释,对极抽象或关联偏远的概念的理解有些困难
4	中度	经常运用具体化的思维模式,对大多数谚语和某些分类理解有困难,倾向于被功能性和显著特征所迷惑
5	偏重	以具体化的思维模式为主,对理解大多数谚语和许多分类有困难
6	重度	无法领会任何谚语或比喻的抽象意义,仅能对最简单的相似事例作公式化的分类,思维空洞贫乏,或固定在功能性方面、显著特征和个人特质的解释
7	极重度	只会使用具体化的思维模式,显示对谚语、一般隐喻或明喻及最简单的分类无法理解,甚至不会用显著的和功能性的特征作为分类的依据。本分级可适用于因显著认知功能缺损而无法与检查者进行最低限度交流的情况

◆ 所问的相似性问题和谚语解释类问题应由易到难,包括易、中、难 3 个层次,且必须是患者所听说过的,否则不算。建议按患者实际回答问题的情况做出评分,检查用语参见 SCI-PANSS 中的 N5 部分。

N6. 交谈缺乏自发性和流畅性

交谈的正常流畅性下降,伴有淡漠、缺乏意志、防卫,或认知缺损,患者表现在语言交流过程的流畅性和创造性下降。

评分依据:会谈中观察患者的认知言语过程。

	评分	标　　准
1	无	定义不适用于该患者
2	很轻	症状可疑,但可能是正常范围的上限
3	轻度	交谈显示很少有主动性,患者的回答简短且不加修饰,需要会谈者给予直接的和引导性的问题
4	中度	患者交谈缺乏自然流畅,显得不顺畅或停顿,在交谈过程中,经常需要对问题加以引导,以诱导出充分的回答
5	偏重	患者表现明显的缺乏自发性及坦率,回答会谈者提问时仅用一个或两个简短的句子
6	重度	患者的回答仅局限于几个单字或短语,以回避或缩短交谈(如"我不知道","我没空说。"),使交谈发生严重困难,且毫无效果
7	极重度	语言的流出最多局限于偶然的吃语,使交谈无法进行

◆ 主要指思维贫乏,或情感障碍,或意志障碍,或认知缺损引起的语言量的减少。思维散漫所致的语言不流畅不包括在此。

◆ 若谈话显示很少有主动性、需要评分员给予引导性的回答问题,则评为轻度(3 分)。

◆ 不稳定或谈话有停顿的,且需要经常给予引导性的回答问题,则评为中度(4 分)。

N7. Stereotyped thinking

Decreased fluidity, spontaneity, and flexibility of thinking, as evidenced in rigid, repetitious, or barren thought content.

Basis for rating: cognitive-verbal processes observed during the interview.

	Rating	Criteria
1	Absent	Definition does not apply
2	Minimal	Questionable pathology; may be at the upper extreme of normal limits
3	Mild	Some rigidity shown in attitudes or beliefs. Patient may refuse to consider alternative positions or have difficulty in shifting from one idea to another
4	Moderate	Conversation revolves around a recurrent theme, resulting in difficulty in shifting to a new topic
5	Moderate Severe	Thinking is rigid and repetitious to the point that, despite the interviewer's efforts, conversation is limited to only two or three dominating topics
6	Severe	Uncontrolled repetition of demands, statements, ideas, or questions which severely impairs conversation
7	Extreme	Thinking, behavior, and conversation are dominated by constant repetition of fixed ideas or limited phrases, leading to gross rigidity, inappropriateness, and restrictiveness of patient's communication

三 —— **General Psychopathology Scale (G)**

G1. Somatic concern

Physical complaints or beliefs about bodily illness or malfunctions. This may range from a vague sense of ill being to clear-cut delusions of catastrophic physical disease.

Basis for rating: thought content expressed in the interview.

	Rating	Criteria
1	Absent	Definition does not apply
2	Minimal	Questionable pathology; may be at the upper extreme of normal limits
3	Mild	Distinctly concerned about health or somatic issues, as evidenced by occasional questions and desire for reassurance
4	Moderate	Complains about poor health or bodily malfunction, but there is no delusional conviction, and over-concern can be allayed by reassurance
5	Moderate Severe	Patient expresses numerous or frequent complaints about physical illness or bodily malfunction, or else patient reveals one or two clear-cut delusions involving these themes but is not preoccupied by them
6	Severe	Patient is preoccupied by one or a few clear-cut delusions about physical disease or organic malfunction, but affect is not fully immersed in these themes, and thoughts can be diverted by the interviewer with some effort
7	Extreme	Numerous and frequently reported somatic delusions, or only a few somatic delusions of a catastrophic nature, which totally dominate the patient's affect and thinking

N7. 刻板思维

思维的流畅性、自发性和灵活性下降,表现在刻板、重复或思维内容空洞。

评分依据:会谈中观察患者认知言语过程。

	评分	标 准
1	无	定义不适用于该患者
2	很轻	症状可疑,但可能是正常范围的上限
3	轻度	态度或信念有些僵化,患者可能拒绝考虑另一种见解,或难以从一种观点改变成另一种观点
4	中度	交谈围绕着一个重复的主题,导致改变话题困难
5	偏重	患者思维刻板及重复,尽管会谈者做出努力,交谈仍仅局限于二三个受限的主题
6	重度	患者无法控制地重复要求、声明、观点或问题,严重地妨碍交谈
7	极重度	患者思维、行为和交谈被不断重复的牢固的观点或有限的短语所支配,导致患者的交流明显刻板、不恰当,并受到限制

三 ···· 一般精神病理量表

G1. 关注身体健康

诉说躯体不适或坚信有躯体疾病或功能失常,其范围从模糊的患病感到明确的身患重病的妄想。

评分依据:会谈中患者表达的思维内容。

	评分	标 准
1	无	定义不适用于该患者
2	很轻	症状可疑,但可能是正常范围的上限
3	轻度	患者明显地关心自身健康或身体问题,偶尔会提出问题并希望得到保证
4	中度	主诉健康不佳或身体功能失常,但没有达到妄想的确信无疑,患者的过度关心可通过给予保证而减轻
5	偏重	患者大量或频繁地主诉患躯体疾病或身体功能失常,或显露一两个关于这些主题的明显妄想,但尚未被其占据
6	重度	患者思维被一个或几个明显的关于躯体疾病或器质性功能失常的妄想所占据,但情感尚未完全陷入其中,其思维经会谈者的努力能有所转移
7	极重度	大量而频繁地诉说躯体妄想,或是一些灾难性的躯体妄想,妄想完全支配患者的情感和思维

◆ G1 涉及对躯体的关注,可有或没有现实根据。

◆ 躯体妄想评≥5 分。

G2. Anxiety

Subjective experience of nervousness，worry，apprehension，or restlessness，ranging from excessive concern about the present or future to feelings of panic.

Basis for rating： verbal report during the course of interview and corresponding phyical manifestations.

	Rating	Criteria
1	Absent	Definition does not apply
2	Minimal	Questionable pathology；may be at the upper extreme of normal limits
3	Mild	Expresses some worry, over-concern, or subjective restlessness, but no somatic and behavioral consequences are reported or evidenced
4	Moderate	Patient reports distinct symptoms of nervousness, which are reflected in mild physical manifestations such as fine hand tremor and excessive perspiration
5	Moderate Severe	Patient reports serious problems of anxiety, which have significant physical and behavioral consequences, such as marked tension, poor concentration, palpitations, or impaired sleep
6	Severe	Subjective state of almost constant fear associated with phobias, marked restlessness, or numerous somatic manifestations
7	Extreme	Patient's life is seriously disrupted by anxiety, which is present almost constantly and, at times, reaches panic proportion or is manifested in actual panic attacks

G3. Guilt feelings

Sense of remorse or self blame for real or imagined misdeeds in the past.

Basis for rating： verbal report of guilt feelings during the course of interview and the influence on attitudes and thoughts.

	Rating	Criteria
1	Absent	Definition does not apply
2	Minimal	Questionable pathology；may be at the upper extreme of normal limits
3	Mild	Questioning elicits a vague sense of guilt or self-blame for a minor incident, but the patient clearly is not overly concerned
4	Moderate	Patient expresses distinct concern over his or her responsibility for a real incident in his or her life but is not preoccupied with it, and attitude and behavior are essentially unaffected
5	Moderate Severe	Patient expresses a strong sense of guilt associated with self-deprecation or the belief that he or she deserves punishment. The guilt feelings may have a delusional basis, may be volunteered spontaneously, may be a source of preoccupation and/or depressed mood, and cannot be allayed readily by the interviewer
6	Severe	Strong ideas of guilt take on a delusional quality and lead to an attitude of hopelessness or worthlessness. The patient believes he or she should receive harsh sanctions for the misdeeds and may even regard his or her current life situation as such punishment
7	Extreme	Patient's life is dominated by unstable delusions of guilt, for which he or she feels deserving of drastic punishment, such as life imprisonment, torture, or death. There may be associated suicidal thoughts or attribution of others' problems to one's own past misdeeds

G2. 焦虑

主观体验到神经紧张、担忧、恐惧或坐立不安,其范围从对现在或将来的过分关心到惊恐的感觉。

评分依据:会谈中患者的语言表达和相应的躯体表现。

	评分	标　　准
1	无	定义不适用于该患者
2	很轻	症状可疑,但可能是正常范围的上限
3	轻度	患者表示有些担忧、过度关心或主观的坐立不安,但没有诉说或表现出相应的躯体症状和行为
4	中度	患者诉说有明显的神经紧张症状,并反映出轻微的躯体症状,如手的细微震颤和过度出汗
5	偏重	患者诉说有严重的焦虑问题,具有显著的躯体症状和行为表现,如明显的肌肉紧张、注意力下降、心悸或睡眠障碍
6	重度	几乎持续感受到害怕并伴有恐惧,患者有明显的坐立不安,或有许多躯体症状
7	极重度	患者的生活严重地被焦虑困扰,焦虑几乎持续存在,有时达到惊恐的程度或表现为惊恐性发作

G3. 自罪感

为过去真实或想象的过失而后悔或自责的感觉。

评分依据:会谈中患者语言表达的自罪感及对态度和思维的影响。

	评分	标　　准
1	无	定义不适用于该患者
2	很轻	症状可疑,但可能是正常范围的上限
3	轻度	询问时引出患者对微小事件的模糊的内疚或自责感,但患者显然并不过分在意
4	中度	患者明确表示在意他对过去发生的一件真实事件的责任,但并未被其占据,态度和行为基本未受影响
5	偏重	患者表示出强烈的罪恶感,伴有自我责难或认为自己应受惩罚。罪恶感可能有妄想基础,可能自发形成,可能来源于某种先占观念和(或)抑郁心境,且不易被测试者缓解
6	重度	带有妄想性质的强烈的罪恶观念,导致出现绝望感或无价值感,患者认为应该为其过失受到严厉制裁,甚至认为他现在的生活处境就是这种惩罚
7	极重度	患者的生活被反复无常的罪恶妄想所支配,感到自己应受严厉的惩罚,如终身监禁、酷刑或处死,可能伴有自杀观念,或将他人的问题归咎于自己过去的过失

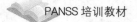
G4. Tension

Overt physical manifestations of fear, anxiety, and agitation, such as stiffness, tremor, profuse sweating, and restlessness.

Basis for rating: verbal report attesting to anxiety and, thereupon, the severity of physical manifestations of tension observed during the interview.

	Rating	Criteria
1	Absent	Definition does not apply
2	Minimal	Questionable pathology; may be at the upper extreme of normal limits
3	Mild	Posture and movements indicate slight apprehensiveness, such as minor rigidity, occasional restlessness, shifting of position, or fine rapid hand tremor
4	Moderate	A clearly nervous appearance emerges from various manifestations, such as fidgety behavior, obvious hand tremor, excessive perspiration, or nervous mannerisms
5	Moderate Severe	Pronounced tension is evidenced by numerous manifestations, such as nervous shaking, profuse sweating, and restlessness, but conduct in the interview is not significantly affected
6	Severe	Pronounced tension to the point that interpersonal interactions are disrupted. The patient, for example, may be constantly fidgeting, unable to sit still for long, or show hyperventilation
7	Extreme	Marked tension is manifested by signs of panic or gross motor acceleration, such as rapid restless pacing and inability to remain seated for longer than a minute, which makes sustained conversation not possible

G5. Mannerisms and posturing

Unnatural movements or posture as characterized by an awkward, stilted, disorganized, or bizarre appearance.

Basis for rating: observation of physical manifestations during the course of interview as well as reports from primary care workers or family.

	Rating	Criteria
1	Absent	Definition does not apply
2	Minimal	Questionable pathology; may be at the upper extreme of normal limits
3	Mild	Slight awkwardness in movements or minor rigidity of posture
4	Moderate	Movements are notably awkward or disjointed, or an unnatural posture is maintained for brief periods
5	Moderate Severe	Occasional bizarre rituals or contorted posture are observed, or an abnormal position is sustained for extended periods
6	Severe	Frequent repetition of bizarre rituals, mannerisms, or stereotyped movements, or a contorted posture is sustained for extended periods
7	Extreme	Functioning is seriously impaired by virtually constant involvement in ritualistic, manneristic, or stereotyped movements or by an unnatural fixed posture which is sustained most of the time

G4. 紧张

因恐惧、焦虑和激越而表现明显的躯体症状,如僵直、震颤、大量出汗和坐立不安。

评分依据:会谈中患者语言表达的焦虑及紧张的躯体表现的严重程度。

	评分	标　准
1	无	定义不适用于该患者
2	很轻	症状可疑,但可能是正常范围的上限
3	轻度	姿势和动作表现出轻微的担忧,如轻度僵硬,偶尔坐立不安,变换姿势或手部轻微快速震颤
4	中度	患者明显地表现为多种紧张症状,如局促不安、明显的手部颤抖、过度出汗,或紧张性作态
5	偏重	显著的紧张表现为许多症状,如紧张性颤抖、大量出汗和坐立不安,但会谈的过程并未受到明显的影响
6	重度	显著的紧张表现妨碍人际交往,如持续的局促不安、无法静坐或过度换气
7	极重度	明显的紧张表现为惊恐症状或显著的动作加速,如快速地来回走动和无法静坐超过 1 分钟,使会谈无法进行

◆ 条目 G2(焦虑)是评估焦虑的主观体验(包括对焦虑相关性躯体症状的主观体验),而条目 G4(紧张)聚焦于在访谈中观察到的患者明显的焦虑及相关性躯体表现。

G5. 装相和作态

不自然的动作或姿势,以笨拙、做作、紊乱或古怪表现为特征。

评分依据:会谈中观察患者躯体表现,也可由基层保健工作者或家属提供患者的情况。

	评分	标　准
1	无	定义不适用于该患者
2	很轻	症状可疑,但可能是正常范围的上限
3	轻度	动作有点笨拙或姿势有些僵硬
4	中度	动作明显笨拙或不连贯,或短时间保持一种不自然的姿势
5	偏重	观察到患者偶有古怪的仪式性动作或扭曲的姿势,或长时间保持一种异常的姿势
6	重度	经常重复出现古怪的仪式性动作、装相或刻板动作,或长时间保持一种扭曲的姿势
7	极重度	几乎持续不断的仪式性动作、装相或刻板动作导致功能严重受损,或大部分时间保持一种不自然的固定姿势

G6. Depression

Feelings of sadness, discouragement, helplessness, and pessimism.

Basis for rating: verbal report of depressed mood during the course of interview and its observed influence on attitude and behavior as reported by primary care workers or family.

	Rating	Criteria
1	Absent	Definition does not apply
2	Minimal	Questionable pathology; may be at the upper extreme of normal limits
3	Mild	Expresses some sadness or discouragement only on questioning, but there is no evidence of depression in general attitude or demeanor
4	Moderate	Distinct feelings of sadness or hopelessness, which may be spontaneously divulged, but depressed mood has no major impact on behavior or social functioning, and the patient usually can be cheered up
5	Moderate Severe	Distinctly depressed mood is associated with obvious sadness, pessimism, loss of social interest, psychomotor retardation, and some interference in appetite and sleep. The patient cannot be easily cheered up
6	Severe	Markedly depressed mood is associated with sustained feelings of misery, occasional crying, hopelessness, and worthlessness. In addition, there is major interference in appetite and/or sleep as well as in normal motor and social functions, with possible signs of self-neglect
7	Extreme	Depressive feelings seriously interfere in most major functions. The manifestations include frequent crying, pronounced somatic symptoms, impaired concentration, psychomotor retardation, social disinterest, self-neglect, possible depressive or nihilistic delusions, and/or possible suicidal thoughts or actions

G7. Motor retardation

Reduction in motor activity as reflected in slowing or lessening of movements and speech, diminished responsiveness to stimuli, and reduced body tone.

Basis for rating: manifestations during the course of interview as well as reports by primary care workers or family.

	Rating	Criteria
1	Absent	Definition does not apply
2	Minimal	Questionable pathology; may be at the upper extreme of normal limits
3	Mild	Slight but noticeable diminution in rate of movements and speech. Patient may be somewhat underproductive in conversation and gestures
4	Moderate	Patient is clearly slow in movements, and speech may be characterized by poor productivity, including long response latency, extended pauses, or slow pace
5	Moderate Severe	A marked reduction in motor activity renders communication highly unproductive or delimits functioning in social and occupational situations. Patient can usually be found sitting or lying down
6	Severe	Movements are extremely slow, resulting in a minimum of activity and speech. Essentially the day is spent sitting idly or lying down
7	Extreme	Patient is almost completely immobile and virtually unresponsive to external stimuli

G6. 抑郁

悲伤、沮丧、无助和悲观厌世的感觉。

评分依据： 会谈中患者抑郁心境的言语表达，及对患者态度和行为的影响，也可由基层保健工作者或家属提供患者的状况。

	评分	标　　准
1	无	定义不适用于该患者
2	很轻	症状可疑，但可能是正常范围的上限
3	轻度	只在被问及时患者才表示有些悲伤或沮丧，但总的态度或行为举止没有抑郁表现
4	中度	明显感到悲伤或绝望可能是患者自然流露出来的情绪，但抑郁心境未对行为或社会功能造成重大影响，而且患者通常还能高兴起来
5	偏重	明显感受到患者的抑郁心境，并伴有明显的悲伤、悲观厌世、失去社交兴趣和精神运动迟滞，对食欲和睡眠有些妨碍，患者不易高兴起来
6	重度	明显感受到患者的抑郁心境，并伴有持续的痛苦感，偶尔哭泣、绝望和无价值感；另外，对食欲和(或)睡眠以及正常运动和社会功能有严重妨碍，可能有自我忽视的迹象
7	极重度	抑郁感觉严重妨碍患者大部分主要功能，表现包括经常哭泣，有明显的躯体症状，注意力损害，精神运动迟滞，失去社交兴趣，自我忽视，可能有抑郁或虚无妄想，和(或)可能有自杀意念或行为

G7. 运动迟缓

运动减少，表现在动作和言语的减慢或减少，对刺激的反应减弱及体质变弱。

评分依据： 会谈中患者的表现，也可由基层保健工作者或家属提供患者的状况。

	评分	标　　准
1	无	定义不适用于该患者
2	很轻	症状可疑，但可能是正常范围的上限
3	轻度	轻微但明显的动作和讲话速度减慢，患者在交谈中谈话内容和姿势可能有点不足
4	中度	患者的动作明显减慢，讲话的特点是讲话内容不足，包括反应期延长、停顿延长或语速缓慢
5	偏重	运动活动显著减少，导致交谈内容非常不足，或影响社交和职业功能，常常发现患者呆坐着或躺着
6	重度	动作极其缓慢，导致极少活动和讲话，患者基本上整天呆坐或躺着
7	极重度	患者几乎完全不动，并且对外界刺激毫无反应

◆ 评定时不考虑药物所致 EPS 反应。

◆ 评 4 分(中度)或以上可包括在访谈中观察到的患者讲话内容不足、反应期延长，或停顿延长，或语速缓慢。

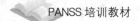

G8. Uncooperativeness

Active refusal to comply with the will of significant others, including the interviewer, hospital staff, or family, which may be associated with distrust, defensiveness, stubbornness, negativism, rejection of authority, hostility, or belligerence.

Basis for rating: interpersonal behavior observed during the course of interview as well as reports by primary care workers or family.

	Rating	Criteria
1	Absent	Definition does not apply
2	Minimal	Questionable pathology; may be at the upper extreme of normal limits
3	Mild	Complies with an attitude of resentment, impatience, or sarcasm. May inoffensively object to sensitive probing during the interview
4	Moderate	Occasional outright refusal to comply with normal social demands, such as making own bed, attending scheduled programs, etc. The patient may project a hostile, defensive, or negative attitude but usually can be worked with
5	Moderate Severe	Patient frequently is incompliant with the demands of his or her milieu and may be characterized by others as an "outcast" or having "a serious attitude problem". Uncooperativeness is reflected in obvious defensiveness or irritability with the interviewer and possible unwillingness to address many questions
6	Severe	Patient is highly uncooperative, negativistic, and possibly also belligerent. Refuses to comply with most social demands and may be unwilling to initiate or conclude the full interview
7	Extreme	Active resistance seriously impacts on virtually all major areas of functioning. Patient may refuse to join in any social activities, tend to personal hygiene, converse with family or staff, and participate even briefly in an interview

G9. Unusual thought content

Thinking characterized by strange, fantastic, or bizarre ideas, ranging from those, which are remote or atypical to those which are distorted, illogical, and patently absurd.

Basis for rating: thought content expressed during the course of interview.

	Rating	Criteria
1	Absent	Definition does not apply
2	Minimal	Questionable pathology; may be at the upper extreme of normal limits
3	Mild	Thought content is somewhat peculiar or idiosyncratic, or familiar ideas are framed in an odd context
4	Moderate	Ideas are frequently distorted and occasionally seem quite bizarre
5	Moderate Severe	Patient expresses many strange and fantastic thoughts (e.g., being the adopted son of a king, being an escapee from death row) or some which are patently absurd (e.g., having hundreds of children, receiving radio messages from outer space through a tooth filling)
6	Severe	Patient expresses many illogical or absurd ideas or some, which have a distinctly bizarre quality (e.g., having three heads, being a visitor from another planet)
7	Extreme	Thinking is replete with absurd, bizarre, and grotesque ideas

G8. 不合作

主动拒绝顺从其他重要人物的意愿,包括会谈者、医务人员或家属,可能伴有不信任、防御、固执、消极、抵制权威、敌对或好斗。

评分依据:会谈中观察患者的人际行为,也可由基层保健工作者或家属提供患者的状况。

	评分	标 准
1	无	定义不适用于该患者
2	很轻	症状可疑,但可能是正常范围的上限
3	轻度	以一种愤恨、不耐烦或讥讽的态度服从。会谈中可能婉转地反对敏感问题
4	中度	偶尔直率地拒绝服从正常的社会要求,如整理自己的床铺,参加安排好的活动等。患者可能表现出敌对、防御或否定的态度,但通常仍可共事
5	偏重	患者经常不遵从周围环境的要求,可能被他人描述为"被遗弃者"或有"严重的态度问题",不合作表现为对测试者明显的防御或易激怒,可能对许多问题不愿回答
6	重度	患者高度不合作、抗拒,而且还可能好斗,拒绝服从大部分社会要求,可能不愿开始或完成整个会谈
7	极重度	主动地抵制,严重影响几乎所有主要的功能领域,患者可能拒绝参加任何社交活动,不注意个人卫生,不与家属或工作人员谈话,或甚至拒绝参与简短的会谈

G9. 不寻常思维内容

思维特征为奇怪、幻想式或荒诞的念头,其范围从离谱或不典型到歪曲的、不合逻辑的和明显荒谬的想法。

评分依据:会谈中患者对有关思维内容的表达。

	评分	标 准
1	无	定义不适用于该患者
2	很轻	症状可疑,但可能是正常范围的上限
3	轻度	思维内容有些奇怪或特异,或熟悉的观念却用在古怪的语境文中
4	中度	观念经常被歪曲,偶尔显得非常古怪
5	偏重	患者表达许多奇怪的幻想的思维内容(如是国王的养子,是死亡名单的逃脱者)或一些明显荒谬的想法(如有几百个子女,通过牙齿填充物收到来自外太空的无线电信息)
6	重度	患者表达许多不合逻辑的或荒谬的观念,有些具有非常古怪的性质(如有 3 个脑袋,是外星人)
7	极重度	思维充满荒谬、古怪和怪诞的想法

◆ (3分或 4 分)可反映出患者有古怪的或荒诞的而不一定是妄想性的想法。

G10. Disorientation

Lack of awareness of one's relationship to the milieu, including persons, place, and time, which may be due to confusion or withdrawal.

Basis for rating: responses to interview questions on orientation.

	Rating	Criteria
1	Absent	Definition does not apply
2	Minimal	Questionable pathology; may be at the upper extreme of normal limits
3	Mild	General orientation is adequate but there is some difficulty with specifics. For example, patient knows his or her location but not the street address; knows hospital staff names but not their functions; knows the month but confuses the day of week with an adjacent day; or errs in the date by more than two days. There may be narrowing of interest evidenced by familiarity with the immediate but not extended milieu, such as ability to identify staff but not the Mayor, Governor, or President
4	Moderate	Only partial success in recognizing persons, places, and time. For example, patient knows he or she is in a hospital but not its name; knows the name of his or her city but not the borough or district, knows the name of his or her primary therapist but not many other direct care workers; knows the year and season but is not sure of the month
5	Moderate Severe	Considerable failure in recognizing persons, place, and time. Patient has only a vague notion of where he or she is and seems unfamiliar with most people in his or her milieu. He or she may identify the year correctly or nearly so but not know the current month, day of week, or even the season
6	Severe	Marked failure in recognizing persons, place, and time. For example, patient has no knowledge of his or her whereabouts; confuses the date by more than one year; can name only one or two individuals in his or her current life
7	Extreme	Patient appears completely disoriented with regard to persons, place, and time. There is gross confusion or total ignorance about one's location, the current year, and even the most familiar people, such as parents, spouse, friends, and primary therapist

G11. Poor attention

Failure in focused alertness manifested by poor concentration, distractibility from internal and external stimuli, and difficulty in harnessing, sustaining, or shifting focus to new stimuli.

Basis for rating: manifestations during the course of interview.

	Rating	Criteria
1	Absent	Definition does not apply
2	Minimal	Questionable pathology; may be at the upper extreme of normal limits
3	Mild	Limited concentration evidenced by occasional vulnerability to distraction or faltering attention toward the end of the interview
4	Moderate	Conversation is affecd by the tendency to be easily distracted, difficulty in long sustaining concentration on a given topic, or problems in shifting attention to new topics
5	Moderate Severe	Conversation is seriously hampered by poor concentration, distractibility, and difficulty in shifting focus appropriately
6	Severe	Patient's attention can be harnessed for only brief moments or with great effort, due to marked distraction by internal or external stimuli
7	Extreme	Attention is so disrupted that even brief conversation is not possible

G10. 定向障碍

丧失与环境有关的意识,包括人物、地点和时间,可能由意识混乱或戒断引起。

评分依据:会谈中患者对定向问题的反应。

	评分	标　　准
1	无	定义不适用于该患者
2	很轻	症状可疑,但可能是正常范围的上限
3	轻度	一般的定向尚可,但精确的定向有些困难,如患者知道他在何地,但不知道确切地址;知道医院工作人员的名字,但不知道他们的职能;知道月份,但星期几搞错1天;或日期相差2天以上。可能有兴趣范围狭窄,表现为只熟悉身边的环境,但不知道外围的环境,如能认识工作人员,但不认识市长、首脑或总统
4	中度	只能对时间、地点、人物部分定向,如患者知道他在医院里,但不知道医院的名称;知道他所在的城市名称,但不知道村镇或行政区的名称;知道他主治人员的名字,但不知道其他直接照料者的名字;知道年份和季节,但不知道确切的月份
5	偏重	人物、时间、地点的定向力大部分受损,患者只有一些模糊的概念,如他在何处,似乎对环境中的大多数人都感觉陌生,可能会正确或接近地说出年份,但月份、星期几或甚至季节都不知道
6	重度	人物、时间、地点定向力明显丧失。如:患者不知道身在何处,对日期的误差超过1年;仅能说出当前生活中一两个人名
7	极重度	患者完全丧失人物、地点、时间定向力,严重混淆或全然不知自己身在何处,现在的年份,甚至最熟悉的人,如父母、配偶、朋友和主治人员

◆ 不限于意识障碍所致的定向障碍;若各分级标准间有重叠,按重度的计分。

G11. 注意障碍

警觉集中障碍,表现为注意力不集中,受内外刺激而分散注意力,以及在驾驭、保持或转移注意力至新刺激时存在困难。

评分依据:会谈中患者的表现。

	评分	标　　准
1	无	定义不适用于该患者
2	很轻	症状可疑,但可能是正常范围的上限
3	轻度	注意力集中受限,偶尔容易分心或在会谈将结束时显得注意力不集中
4	中度	会谈因注意力容易分散的倾向而受到影响,难以长时间将注意力集中在一个主题上,或难以将注意力转向新的主题
5	偏重	会谈因为注意力不集中、分散和难以适当地转换注意点而受到严重影响
6	重度	患者的注意力由于受内在的或外部的刺激而明显分散,注意力仅能维持片刻或须做很大努力
7	极重度	注意力严重障碍,以致简短的交谈都无法进行

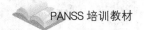

G12. Lack of judgment and insight

Impaired awareness or understanding of one's own psychiatric condition and life situation. This is evidenced by failure to recognize past or present psychiatric illness or symptoms, denial of need for psychiatric hospitalization or treatment, decisions characterized by poor anticipation of consequences, and unrealistic short-term and long-range planning.

Basis for rating: thought content expressed during the interview.

	Rating	Criteria
1	Absent	Definition does not apply
2	Minimal	Questionable pathology; may be at the upper extreme of normal limits
3	Mild	Recognizes having a psychiatric disorder but clearly underestimates its seriousness, the implications for treatment, or the importance of taking measures to avoid relapse. Future planning may be poorly conceived
4	Moderate	Patient shows only a vague or shallow recognition of illness. There may be fluctuations in acknowledgment of being ill or little awareness of major symptoms, which are present, such as delusions, disorganized thinking, suspiciousness, and social withdrawal. The patient may rationalize the need for treatment in terms of its relieving lesser symptoms, such as anxiety, tension, and sleep difficulty
5	Moderate Severe	Acknowledges past but not present psychiatric disorder. If challenged, the patient may concede the presence of some unrelated or insignificant symptoms, which tend to be explained away by gross misinterpretation or delusional thinking. The need for psychiatric treatment similarly goes unrecognized
6	Severe	Patient denies ever having had a psychiatric disorder. He or she disavows the presence of any psychiatric symptoms in the past or present and, though compliant, denies the need for treatment and hospitalization
7	Extreme	Emphatic denial of past and present psychiatric illness. Current hospitalization and treatment are given a delusional interpretation (e.g., as punishment for misdeeds, as persecution by tormentors, etc.), and the patient may thus refuse to cooperate with therapists, medication, or other aspects of treatment

G13. Disturbance of volition

Disturbance in the willful initiation, sustenance, and control of one's thoughts, behavior, movements, and speech.

Basis for rating: thought content and behavior manifested in the course of interview.

	Rating	Criteria
1	Absent	Definition does not apply
2	Minimal	Questionable pathology; may be at the upper extreme of normal limits
3	Mild	There is evidence of some indecisiveness in conversation and thinking, which may impede verbal and cognitive processes to a minor extent
4	Moderate	Patient is often ambivalent and shows clear difficulty in reaching decisions. Conversation may be marred by alteration in thinking, and in consequence verbal and cognitive functioning are clearly impaired
5	Moderate Severe	Disturbance of volition interferes in thinking as well as behavior. Patient shows pronounced indecision that impedes the initiation and continuation of social and motor activities, and which also may be evidenced in halting speech
6	Severe	Disturbance of volition interferes in the execution of simple, automatic motor functions, such as dressing and grooming, and markedly affects speech
7	Extreme	Almost complete failure of volition is manifested by gross inhibition of movement and speech, resulting in immobility and/or mutism

G12. 判断和自知力缺乏

对自身精神状况和生活处境的认识或理解受损,表现在不能认识过去或现在的精神疾病或症状,否认需要在精神科住院或治疗,所做决定的特点是对后果的预期很差,及不切实际的短期和长期计划。

评分依据:会谈中患者对有关思维内容的表达。

	评分	标 准
1	无	定义不适用于该患者
2	很轻	症状可疑,但可能是正常范围的上限
3	轻度	认识到有某种精神障碍,但明显低估其严重性、治疗的意义或采取措施以避免复发的重要性,对未来计划的构想力可能较差
4	中度	患者表现为对疾病只有模糊或肤浅的认识,对于承认患病的认识动摇不定,或对存在的主要症状很少认识,如妄想、思维混乱、猜疑和社交退缩,患者可能将需要治疗理解为减轻一些较轻的症状,如焦虑、紧张和睡眠困难
5	偏重	认识到过去但不是现在有精神障碍,如被质疑,患者可能勉强承认一些无关的或不重要的症状,并倾向于以完全曲解的解释或妄想性思维来加以开脱,同样,认为不需要精神治疗
6	重度	患者否认曾患精神障碍,患者否认过去或现在存在任何精神症状,尽管尚能顺从,但否认需要治疗和住院
7	极重度	断然否认过去和现在存在精神疾病,对目前的住院和治疗给予妄想性的解释(如因过失而受惩罚、被人迫害等),患者因此拒绝与治疗者配合,拒绝药物或其他治疗

◆ 评估此条目只考虑患者对自己的精神病病情和生活状况的认识或理解。
◆ 此条目并非更广义地评估针对评估期间患者总体的信念和行为的自知力。

G13. 意志障碍

意志的产生、维持,及对思维、行为、动作、语言的控制障碍。

评分依据:会谈中患者的思维内容和行为表现。

	评分	标 准
1	无	定义不适用于该患者
2	很轻	症状可疑,但可能是正常范围的上限
3	轻度	患者的谈话和思维有些犹豫不决,轻度妨碍言语和认知过程
4	中度	患者经常出现矛盾症状,做决定有明显的困难,交谈可因思维的变化不定而受影响,言语和认知功能明显受损
5	偏重	意志障碍妨碍思维及行为,患者表现为严重的犹豫不决,妨碍社会和动作活动的产生和持续,也可能表现为言语停顿
6	重度	意志障碍妨碍执行简单的、自主的动作功能,如穿衣和梳理,明显地影响言语功能
7	极重度	意志几乎完全丧失,表现为严重的运动和语言抑制,导致不动和(或)缄默

◆ 指矛盾意志,犹豫不决的程度。

G14. Poor impulse control

Disordered regulation and control of action on inner urges, resulting in sudden, unmodulated, arbitrary, or misdirected discharge of tension and emotions without concern about consequences.

Basis for rating: behavior during the course of interview and reported by primary care workers or family.

	Rating	Criteria
1	Absent	Definition does not apply
2	Minimal	Questionable pathology; may be at the upper extreme of normal limits
3	Mild	Patient tends to be easily angered and frustrated when facing stress or denied gratification but rarely acts on impulse
4	Moderate	Patient gets angered and verbally abusive with minimal provocation. May be occasionally threatening, destructive, or have one or two episodes involving physical confrontation or a minor brawl
5	Moderate Severe	Patient exhibits repeated impulsive episodes involving verbal abuse, destruction of property, or physical threats. There may be one or two episodes involving serious assault, for which the patient requires isolation, physical restraint, or p. r. n. sedation
6	Severe	Patient frequently is impulsively aggressive, threatening, demanding, and destructive, without any apparent consideration of consequences. Shows assaultive behavior and may also be sexually offensive and possibly respond behaviorally to hallucinatory commands
7	Extreme	Patient exhibits homicidal attacks, sexual assaults, repeated brutality, or self-destructive behavior. Requires constant direct supervision or external constraints because of inability to control dangerous impulses

G15. Preoccupation

Absorption with internally generated thoughts and feelings and with autistic experiences to the detriment of reality orientation and adaptive behavior.

Basis for rating: interpersonal behavior observed during the course of interview.

	Rating	Criteria
1	Absent	Definition does not apply
2	Minimal	Questionable pathology; may be at the upper extreme of normal limits
3	Mild	Excessive involvement with personal needs or problems, such that conversation veers back to egocentric themes and there is diminished concern exhibited toward others
4	Moderate	Patient occasionally appears self-absorbed, as if daydreaming or involved with internal experiences, which interferes with communication to a minor extent
5	Moderate Severe	Patient often appears to be engaged in autistic experiences, as evidenced by behaviors that significantly intrude on social and communicational functions, such as the presence of a vacant stare, muttering or talking to oneself, or involvement with stereotyped motor patterns
6	Severe	Marked preoccupation with autistic experiences, which seriously delimits concerntration, ability to converse, and orientation to the milieu. The patient frequently may be observed smiling, laughing, muttering, talking, or shouting to himself or herself
7	Extreme	Gross absorption with autistic experiences, which profoundly affects all major realms of behavior. The patient constantly may be responding verbally and behaviorally to hallucinations and show little awareness of other people or the external milieu

G14. 冲动控制障碍

对内在冲动反应的调节和控制障碍,导致不顾后果的、突然的、无法调节的、肆意的或误导的紧张和情绪的宣泄。

评分依据: 会谈中观察患者行为,及由基层保健工作者或家属提供的患者情况。

	评分	标　　准
1	无	定义不适用于该患者
2	很轻	症状可疑,但可能是正常范围的上限
3	轻度	当面对应激或不如意时,患者容易出现愤怒和受挫感,但很少冲动行事
4	中度	患者对轻微的挑衅就会愤怒和谩骂,可能偶尔出现威胁、破坏或一两次身体冲突或程度较轻的吵架
5	偏重	患者反复出现冲动,包括谩骂、毁物或身体威胁,可能有一两次严重的攻击,以致患者需要隔离、身体约束或必要时给予镇静剂
6	重度	患者经常不计后果地出现攻击、威胁、强人所难和破坏性行为,表现出攻击行为并可能是性攻击,可能为对幻听命令的行为反应
7	极重度	患者出现致命的攻击、性侵犯、反复的残暴行为或自残行为;因不能控制其危险性冲动而需要不断的直接监管或外部约束

G15. 先占观念

专注于内在产生的思维和感觉。因内向性体验而损害现实定向和适应性行为。

评分依据: 会谈中观察其人际行为。

	评分	标　　准
1	无	定义不适用于该患者
2	很轻	症状可疑,但可能是正常范围的上限
3	轻度	过分关注个人需要或问题,使会谈转向自我中心的主题,对他人缺乏关心
4	中度	患者偶尔表现自我专注,好像在做白日梦或关注内在体验,轻度妨碍交往
5	偏重	患者常表现为专注于内向性体验,明显影响社交和沟通功能,如出现目光呆滞、喃喃自语或自言自语,或出现刻板的动作模式
6	重度	明显沉浸于内向性体验,使注意力、交谈能力及对环境的定向力严重受限,患者经常一个人微笑、大笑、喃喃自语、自言自语或冲自己大叫
7	极重度	严重地专注于内心体验,极度影响所有重要的行为,患者不断地对幻觉做出言语和行为反应,很少觉察到他人或外部环境

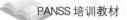

G16. Active social avoidance

Diminished social involvement associated with unwarranted fear, hostility, or distrust.

Basis for rating: reports of social functioning by primary care workers or family.

	Rating	Criteria
1	Absent	Definition does not apply
2	Minimal	Questionable pathology; may be at the upper extreme of normal limits
3	Mild	Patient seems ill at ease in the presence of others and prefers to spend time alone, although he or she participates in social functions when required
4	Moderate	Patient grudgingly attends all or most social activities but may need to be persuaded or may terminate prematurely on account of anxiety, suspiciousness, or hostility
5	Moderate Severe	Patient fearfully or angrily keeps away from many social interactions despite others' efforts to engage him. Tends to spend unstructured time alone
6	Severe	Patient participates in very few social activities because of fear, hostility, or distrust. When approached, the patient shows a strong tendency to break off interactions, and generally he or she appears to isolate himself or herself from others
7	Extreme	Patient cannot be engaged in social activities because of pronounced fears, hostility, or persecutory delusions. To the extent possible, he or she avoids all interactions and remains isolated from others

四 ···· **Supplementary Items for the Aggression Risk Profile**

S1. Anger

Subjective state of displeasure and irritation directed at others.

Basis for rating: verbal report of angry feelings during the course of the interview and, thereupon, corresponding hostile behaviors observed during the interview or noted from reports by primary care workers or family.

	Rating	Criteria
1	Absent	Definition does not apply
2	Minimal	Questionable pathology; may be at the upper extreme of normal limits
3	Mild	Expresses some irritation or ill feelings toward others but, otherwise, shows no emotional or behavioral signs of anger
4	Moderate	Presents an overtly angry exterior, but temper remains under control
5	Moderate Severe	Patient appears highly irritable, and anger is vented through frequently raised voice, occasional verbal abuse, or thinly veiled threats
6	Severe	Patient appears highly irritable, and anger is vented through repeated verbal abuse, overt threats, or destructiveness
7	Extreme	An explosive level of anger is evidenced by physical abuse directed or attempted at others

G16. 主动回避社交

由于无根据的恐惧、敌意或不信任而减少社交参与。

评分依据： 由基层保健工作者或家属提供的患者社交功能状况。

	评分	标　　准
1	无	定义不适用于该患者
2	很轻	症状可疑，但可能是正常范围的上限
3	轻度	患者在别人面前似乎显得不自在，并且喜欢独自消磨时光，尽管他（她）在要求下仍会参加社交活动
4	中度	患者非常勉强地参加所有或大部分社交活动，但可能需要劝说，或可能因焦虑、猜疑或敌意而中止参与
5	偏重	尽管他人努力邀请他，患者仍因恐惧或愤怒而远离许多社会交往，倾向于独自消磨空闲时间
6	重度	患者因恐惧、敌意或不信任而极少参加社交活动。当他人接近时，患者表现出强烈的中止交往的倾向，并且他（她）通常表现出离群索居
7	极重度	患者因极度恐惧、敌意或被害妄想而不参加社交活动，他（她）尽可能回避所有的交往并离群索居

◆ 与 N4 的区分点为社交活动的参与减少是与无根据的恐惧、敌意或不信任有明显联系，是基于他人观察患者所得到的情况。

◆ 因此，此条目的评定说明社交回避是因恐惧、敌意或不信任促成的，而不是因淡漠或缺乏意志力所致。

四　攻击危险性补充项目

S1. 愤怒

主观状态为指向他人的不悦和激惹。

评分依据： 会谈中感觉到患者愤怒的言语表达，及由此观察到的相应敌对行为，或由基层保健工作者或家属提供的患者状况。

	评分	标　　准
1	无	定义不适用于该患者
2	很轻	症状可疑，但可能是正常范围的上限
3	轻度	表达对他人有些激惹或反感，但没有愤怒的情绪或行为表现
4	中度	存在明显的愤怒外表，但脾气仍可控制
5	偏重	患者表现高度激惹，其愤怒通过频繁地提高声音、偶尔的谩骂或稍加掩饰的威胁来发泄
6	重度	患者表现高度激惹，其愤怒通过反复的谩骂、明显的威胁或破坏行为来发泄
7	极重度	愤怒的爆发表现为直接或企图对他人进行人身攻击

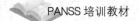

S2. Difficulty in delaying gratification

Demanding, insistent that needs be satisfied immediately, and noticeably upset when fulfillment of needs or desires is delayed.

Basis for rating: observation of behavior during the course of the interview as well as reports from primary care workers or family.

	Rating	Criteria
1	Absent	Definition does not apply
2	Minimal	Questionable pathology; may be at the upper extreme of normal limits
3	Mild	Patient is occasionally demanding and impatient but settles down quickly when spoken to
4	Moderate	Demanding behavior occurs more than just occasionally or else has an insistent quality that makes the patient a "nuisance". No outbursts of hostility, however, typically follow, and the patient ordinarily can be managed without difficulty
5	Moderate Severe	Demanding behavior is both frequent and persistent, resulting in occasional confrontations with other patients, staff, or family. As a rule, however, the patient regains control without serious incident
6	Severe	Patient gets seriously upset whenever needs or demands are not met immediately. Explosive or violent behavior may once or twice ensue, and loss of control is an ever-present possibility
7	Extreme	The failure to instantly cater to the patient's needs or demands tends to provoke explosive, violent, or impulsive behavior. Close supervision is typically required

S3. Affective lability

Emotional expressions are unstable, fluctuating, inappropriate, and/or poorly controlled.

Basis for rating: affective state observed during the course of the interview.

	Rating	Criteria
1	Absent	Definition does not apply
2	Minimal	Questionable pathology; may be at the upper extreme of normal limits
3	Mild	Some incongruous affective responses are observed or a few unexplained shifts in emotional tone may occur
4	Moderate	Affect is frequently incongruent with thoughts (e. g. , inappropriate silliness, anger, or worry), or there are several radical changes in emotional tone during the course of the interview
5	Moderate Severe	Emotional expressions are highly unstable and occasionally seem beyond the patient's control. The affective picture may show sudden shifts to the extremes, with generally poor modulation
6	Severe	Emotions appear to be uncontrolled during most of the interview and may be dominated by autistic or irrelevant stimuli. The affective state takes on a fleeting quality, with peculiar or kaleidoscopic changes. Primitive emotional discharge, e. g. , displays of ecstasy or rage, may be seen
7	Extreme	Patient seems to lack any control over his or her emotional state, which fluctuates freely in response to inappropriate external or internal events. Extreme emotional states, such as excitement or fury, at times dominate

S2. 延迟满足困难

强人所难,坚持立即满足其要求,当需要或渴望被延迟满足时,表现出明显烦乱。

评分依据:会谈中观察其行为,或由基层保健工作者或家属提供患者状况。

	评分	标　　准
1	无	定义不适用于该患者
2	很轻	症状可疑,但可能是正常范围的上限
3	轻度	患者偶有强人所难或不耐烦,但经劝说后能很快平静下来
4	中度	强人所难的行为增多,或带有坚持的特点,使患者成为一个"讨厌的人",但通常没有紧跟着的敌对情绪爆发,一般易于管理
5	偏重	强人所难的行为经常出现且坚持不变,导致偶尔与其他患者、工作人员或家属发生冲突,通常患者能恢复控制,不发生严重事件
6	重度	当需求未被立即满足时,患者表现极为烦乱,随即可发生1～2次暴力行为,随时都可能失去控制
7	极重度	无法立即满足患者的需求,易于发生挑衅、暴力或冲动行为,特别需要密切监护

S3. 情感不稳

情绪表达不稳定、波动、不适当和(或)控制不良。

评分依据:会谈中观察患者的情感状态。

	评分	标　　准
1	无	定义不适用于该患者
2	很轻	症状可疑,但可能是正常范围的上限
3	轻度	观察到患者有些不协调的情感反应,或情绪基调出现一些无法解释的变化
4	中度	情感经常与思维不协调(如不恰当的愚蠢、愤怒或担忧)或会谈中患者情绪基调有几次彻底的改变
5	偏重	情绪表达高度不稳,偶尔似乎超出患者的控制,情感表达可能突然出现极端的改变,通常调节不良
6	重度	会谈中大多数时间情绪无法控制,可能被内在的或无关的刺激支配,情感状态有迅速改变的性质,具有奇特的或千变万化的改变,患者可能出现原始的情绪发泄,如狂喜或暴怒
7	极重度	患者对其情绪状态似乎缺乏任何控制,对不适当的外部或内部事件的反应起伏不定,有时被极端的情绪状态如兴奋或暴怒所支配

五 —— PANSS 评定说明

本量表主要用于评定精神分裂症患者的病情严重程度和疗效。研究表明该量表项目间具有高度内部信度和一致性，各份量表 α 系数为 0.73～0.83。一般精神病理量表分半信度指数为 0.80，重测信度指数为 0.77～0.89。

主要包括阳性量表（7 个条目）、阴性量表（7 个条目）和一般精神病理量表（16 个条目），共 30 个条目。评分为 1～7 分，共 7 级。

评定时间窗为通常为过去 7 天（除非特别定义）的症状；若前次访视距今＜7 天，则评定自前次访视距今时间段内的症状。

评估依据需综合项目定义、评分依据和分级标准三要素，评估每一个症状的有无、出现频度、严重度、症状对行为的影响，尽可能地对每一个要素逐字理解。确定最高一级的严重度评定，不需要符合所有内容；给出一个 1 周内合理的**最高分数**，而不是平均分数。信息来源包括现场访谈时所收集的资料（言语或非言语），及从知情者那里所收集到的过去 1 周的症状。一次访谈评定需 30～40 分钟的时间。

有 6 个条目与妄想有关：P1 妄想；P5 夸大；P6 猜疑或被害感；G1 担心身体健康；G3 罪恶观念；G9 不寻常思维内容。P1 着眼于妄想的数量和系统性；G9 着眼于妄想的怪异性；P5、P6、G1 和 G3 则依妄想的内容评定。

P6 猜疑或被害感是评定可能以防卫行为反映出来的被害妄想，G16 主动回避社交是评定可能继发于被害妄想的行为。有显著妄想的患者因为恐惧或不信任感而只参加少数活动，可能在 P6 和 G16 上评分相似；有明显的系统化被害妄想但极少或没有隔绝的患者可能在 P6 上评分高而在 G16 上评分低。

社交少、活动需督促的表现可在 N2 情绪退缩、N4 被动性或淡漠性社交退缩和 G16 主动回避社交评分，但三项的含义不同。N2 评估情绪退缩，除社交外，尚包括个人事务或个人感兴趣的事，重在个人活动而非人际交往上，原因为不感兴趣；N4 评估淡漠、缺乏精力和缺乏意志，主要指社交活动的不参与，社会活动量的减少；G16 主要指因害怕、恐惧或敌对情绪引起的社交减少，表现为主动回避，而非阴性症状表现。所以社交活动减少，先在 N4 打分，再就其原因分析，评 N2 或 G16。

N1 情感迟钝是指情感的非语言表达，不仅要观察患者的脸部表情，而且还要观察其肢体语言，注意除外药物引起的锥体外系症状；N3 情感交流障碍是 PANSS 中唯一评定对测试者态度的项目；N6 交谈中患者缺乏自发性和流畅性主要指思维贫乏，或情感障碍，或意志障碍，或认知缺损引起的语言量减少。

焦虑与两项有关：G2 焦虑为焦虑的主观体验（包括与焦虑有关的躯体症状的主观体验），若伴有躯体症状，则至少评 4 分或以上；G4 紧张则聚焦于与会谈中观察到的与焦虑有关的明显的躯体表现，包括运动性焦虑；注意排除药物所致 EPS 反应的影响。

冲动打人情况可与 3 个项目有关：P4 兴奋，P7 敌对性和 G14 冲动控制障碍。

G15 先占观念是评定精神分裂症的自闭症状，如有自笑至少评 5 分。

只有 N4 主动回避社交和 G16 主动回避社交仅采用知情者的信息。

应进行有知情者参与的访谈：应由评分员对知情者使用 IQ-PANSS，以收集相关信息。知情者可为：日间活动或康复中心的员工或医院工作人员、家庭成员或与患者有重要且定期接触的其他人。知情者必须可靠。知情者资料中有关患者社会和行为功能的部分，对那些包括来自主要看护者或家人的报告在内作为评分依据的条目来说是必要的。同时需要患者资料和知情者资料的条目为 P1、P3、P4、P5、P6、P7、N2、G5、G6、G7、G8、G14。有 2 个条目的评分只依据知情者资料：N4、G16。

SCI-PANSS

Structured Clinical Interview for the Positive and Negative Syndrome Scale (SCI-PANSS)

Data on "Lack of Spontaneity and Flow of Conversation" (N6), "Poor Roport" (N3), and "Conceptual Disorganization" (P2)

Hi, I'm... We're going to be spending the next 30 to 40 minutes talking about you and your reasons for being here. Maybe you can start out by telling me something about yourself background?

(Instruction to interviewer: Allow at least 5 minutes for a non-directive phrase serving to establish rapport in the context of an overview before proceeding to the specific questions listed below.)

Data on "Anxiety" (G2)

1. Have you been feeling worried or nervous in the past week? _____

IF YES, skip to question 3. IF NO, continue.

2. Would you say that you're usually calm and relaxed? _____

IF YES, skip to question 8. IF NO, continue.

3. What's been making you feel nervous (worried, not calm, not relaxed)? _____

4. Just how nervous (worried, etc.) have you been feeling? _____

5. Have you been shaking at times, or has your heart been racing? _____

6. Do you get into a state of panic? _____

7. Has your sleep, eating, or participation in activities been affected? _____

Data on "Delusions (General)" (P1) and "Unusual Thought Content" (G9)

8. Have things been going well for you? _____

9. Have anything been bothering you lately? _____

10. Can you tell me something about your thoughts on life and its purpose? _____

11. Do you follow a particular philosophy (any special rules, teachings, or religious doctrine)? _____

第三章
SCI-PANSS

阳性和阴性症状量表的定式化临床检查

关于"交谈缺乏自发性和流畅性"(N6)、"情感交流障碍"(N3)和"概念紊乱"(P2)的资料

你好,我是……在随后的30～40分钟里我们将谈及你的一些情况和你来这里的原因。也许你可以先谈谈关于你自己的一些情况。

(给检查者的提示:在对下面所述的特殊问题进行检查之前,应该用至少5分钟的时间进行非定向的会谈,以期有个大致的框架,建立会谈关系。)

关于"焦虑"(G2)的资料

1. 在过去的1周内您是否感到担心或紧张不安? _____

如果回答"是",跳到问题3。如果回答"否",继续。

2. 您是否认为您通常是平静而放松的? _____

如果回答"是",跳到问题8。如果回答"否",继续。

3. 是什么使您感到紧张不安(担心、无法平静、无法放松)? _____

4. 您所感到的紧张不安(担心等)的程度如何? _____

5. 您是否时常出现颤抖,或者是心跳过快? _____

6. 您是否陷入惊恐的状态? _____

7. 您的睡眠、饮食或对活动的参与是否受到了影响? _____

关于"妄想(总体)"(P1)和"不寻常思维内容"(G9)的资料

8. 您的工作生活顺利吗? _____

9. 最近有没有什么事情困扰着您? _____

10. 能不能跟我谈谈您对生活和生活目的的一些看法? _____

11. 您是否遵循某种特定的哲学观点(任何特殊的规则、学说,或宗教教义)? _____

12. Some people tell me they believe in the Devil; what do you think? _____

IF NO (i. e., he/she doesn't believe in the Devil), skip to question 14.

IF YES (i. e., he/she does believe), continue.

13. Can you tell me about this? _____

14. Can you read other people's minds? _____

IF NO, skip to question 16. IF YES, continue.

15. How does that work? _____

16. Can others read your mind? _____

IF NO, skip to question 19. IF YES, continue.

17. How can they do that? _____

18. Is there any reason that someone would want to read your mind? _____

19. Who controls your thoughts? _____

Data on "Suspiciousness/Persecution"（P6）and "Poor Impulse Control"（G14）

20. How do you spend your time these days? _____

21. Do you prefer to be alone? _____

22. Do you join in activities with others? _____

IF YES, skip to question 25. IF NO, continue.

23. Why not? ... Are you afraid of people, or do you dislike them? _____

IF NO, skip to question 26. IF YES, continue.

24. Can you explain? _____

Skip to question 26.

25. Tell me about it. _____

26. Do you have many friends? _____

IF YES, skip to question 30. IF NO, continue.

27. Just a few? _____

IF YES, skip to question 29. IF NO, continue.

28. Any ... Why? _____

Skip to question 32.

29. Why just a few friends? _____

30. Close friends? _____

IF YES, skip to question 32. IF NO, continue.

31. Why not? _____

32. Do you feel that you can trust most people? _____

IF YES, skip to question 34. IF NO, continue.

33. Why not? _____

34. Are there some people in particular who you don't trust? _____

12. 有些人告诉我他们相信魔鬼；您对这一点怎么看的？ _____

如果回答"不"（即他/她不相信魔鬼），跳到问题 14。

如果回答"是"（即他/她相信魔鬼），继续。

13. 您能谈得更具体一些吗？ _____

14. 您能读懂别人的心思吗？ _____

如果回答"不能"，跳到问题 16。如果回答"能"，继续。

15. 那么您是通过什么方式做到这一点的？ _____

16. 其他人能读懂您的心思吗？ _____

如果回答"不能"，跳到问题 19。如果回答"能"，继续。

17. 他们如何做到这一点的？ _____

18. 为什么有人想要读懂您的心思？ _____

19. 谁控制着您的思想？ _____

关于"猜疑、被害"（P6）和"冲动控制障碍"（G14）的资料

20. 您这些天是怎样过的？ _____

21. 您是否宁愿独自待着？ _____

22. 您是否与他人一起参加活动？ _____

如果回答"是"，跳到问题 25。如果回答"否"，继续。

23. 为什么不参与？……您是否害怕他人，或者是您不喜欢他们？ _____

如果回答"不"，跳到问题 26。如果回答"是"，继续。

24. 您能解释一下吗？ _____

跳到问题 26。

25. 跟我谈谈这方面的情况。 _____

26. 您是否有许多朋友？ _____

如果回答"是"，跳到问题 30。如果回答"否"，继续。

27. 几个朋友有吗？ _____

如果回答"是"，跳到问题 29。如果回答"否"，继续。

28. 一个朋友有吗？……为什么？ _____

跳到问题 32。

29. 为什么只有几个朋友？ _____

30. 是亲密的朋友？ _____

如果回答"是"，跳到问题 32。如果回答"否"，继续。

31. 为什么不是？ _____

32. 您是否觉得能够信任大多数人？ _____

如果回答"是"，跳到问题 34。如果回答"否"，继续。

33. 为什么不能？ _____

34. 您是否感到有那么一些人是您不能信任的？ _____

IF NO to question 34 and YES to question 32, skip to question 41.

IF NO to question 34 and NO to question 32, skip to question 36.

IF YES to question 34, continue.

35. Can you tell me who they are? _____

36. Why don't you trust people (or name specific person)? _____

IF "DON'T KNOW" OR "DON'T WANT TO SAY," continue. Otherwise, skip to question 41.

37. Do you have a good reason not to trust …? _____

38. Is there something that … did to you? _____

39. Perhaps something that … might do to you now? _____

IF NO, skip to question 41. IF YES, continue.

40. Can you explain to me? _____

41. Do you get along well with others? _____

IF YES, skip to question 43. IF NO, continue.

42. What's the problem? _____

43. Do you have a quick temper? _____

44. Do you get into fights? _____

IF NO, skip to question 48. IF YES, continue.

45. How do these fights start? _____

46. Tell me about these fights. _____

47. How often does this happen? _____

48. Do you sometimes lose control of yourself? _____

IF NO, skip to question 50. IF YES, continue.

49. What happens when you lose control of yourself? _____

50. Do you like most people? _____

IF YES, skip to question 52. IF NO, continue.

51. Why not? _____

52. Are there perhaps some people who don't like you? _____

IF NO, skip to question 54. IF YES, continue.

53. For what reason? _____

54. Do others talk about you behind your back? _____

IF NO, skip to question 57. IF YES, continue.

55. What do they say about you? _____

56. Why? _____

57. Does anyone ever spy on you or plot against you? _____

58. Do you sometimes feel in danger? _____

IF NO, skip to question 64. IF YES, continue.

如果问题 34 回答"否"，问题 32 回答"是"，跳到问题 41。

如果问题 34 回答"否"，问题 32 回答"否"，跳到问题 36。

如果问题 34 回答"是"，继续。

35. 您能不能告诉我他们是什么人？ _____

36. 您为什么不信任人（或说出某某人的名字）？ _____

如果回答"不知道"或"不想说"，继续。否则，跳到问题 41。

37. 您是否有恰当的理由不信任……？ _____

38. 是否有什么东西……影响您？ _____

39. 也许某些东西……现在正在影响您吧？ _____

如果回答"没有"，跳到问题 41。如果回答"是"，继续。

40. 能够给我解释一下吗？ _____

41. 您和其他人相处得好吗？ _____

如果回答"好"，跳到问题 43。如果回答"不好"，继续。

42. 存在什么问题吗？ _____

43. 您是否是急脾气？ _____

44. 您是否和别人发生冲突？ _____

如果回答"不"，跳到问题 48。如果回答"是"，继续。

45. 这些冲突是怎么开始的？ _____

46. 和我谈谈这些冲突的情况。 _____

47. 这些冲突发生的频率如何？ _____

48. 您是否在某些时候不能控制自己？ _____

如果回答"不是"，跳到问题 50。如果回答"是"，继续。

49. 在您不能控制自己时会发生什么？ _____

50. 您是否喜欢大多数人？ _____

如果回答"是"，跳到问题 52。如果回答"不是"，继续。

51. 为什么不喜欢？ _____

52. 是否可能有些人不喜欢您？ _____

如果回答"不"，跳到问题 54。如果回答"是"，继续。

53. 为什么不喜欢您？ _____

54. 是否有人背地里议论您？ _____

如果回答"没有"，跳到问题 57。如果回答"有"，继续。

55. 他们议论您什么？ _____

56. 为什么议论您？ _____

57. 是否有人窥探您或者阴谋陷害您？ _____

58. 您是否有时感到处于危险中？ _____

如果回答"不"，跳到问题 64。如果回答"是"，继续。

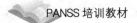
59. Would you say that your life is in danger? _____

60. Is someone thinking of harming you or even perhaps thinking of killing you?

_____

61. Have you gone to the police for help? _____

62. Do you sometimes take matters into your own hands or take action against those who might harm you? _____

IF NO, skip to question 64. IF YES, continue.

63. What have you done? _____

Data on "Hallucinatory Behavior" (P3) and associated delusions

64. Do you once in a while have strange or unusual experiences? _____

65. Sometimes people tell me that they can hear noises or voices inside their head that others can't hear. What about you? _____

IF YES, skip to question 68. IF NO, continue.

66. Do you sometimes receive personal communications from the radio or TV? __

IF YES, skip to question 68. IF NO, continue.

67. From God or the Devil? _____

IF NO, skip to question 83. IF YES, continue.

68. What do you hear? _____

69. Are these as clear and loud as my voice? _____

70. How often do you hear these voices, noises, messages, etc. ? _____

71. Does this happen at a particular time of day or all the time? _____

IF HEARING NOISES ONLY, skip to question 80. IF HEARING VOICES, continue.

72. Can you recognize whose voices these are? _____

73. What do the voices say? _____

74. Are the voices good or bad? _____

75. Pleasant or unpleasant? _____

76. Do the voices interrupt your thinking or your activities? _____

77. Do they sometimes give you orders or instructions? _____

IF NO, skip to question 80. IF YES, continue.

78. For example? _____

79. Do you usually obey these orders (instructions)? _____

80. What do you make of these voices (or noises); where do they really come from? _____

81. Why do you have these experiences? _____

82. Are these normal experiences? _____

83. Do ordinary things sometimes look strange or distorted to you? _____

59. 您是否会说您的生命处于危险中？ _____

60. 是否有人想伤害您或者甚至可能想杀害您？ _____

61. 您是否曾到警察那里寻求帮助？ _____

62. 您是否有时将事情置于您的掌握之中或者对那些可能伤害您的人采取行动？ ___
如果回答"不"，跳到问题64。如果回答"是"，继续。

63. 您是怎么做的？ _____

关于"幻觉性行为"（P3）和相关妄想的资料

64. 您是否曾经出现过奇怪的或不寻常的体验？ _____

65. 有人告诉我他们可以在自己的头脑内听到其他人听不到的噪声或声音。您有这
种感觉吗？ _____
如果回答"有"，跳到问题68。如果回答"没有"，继续。

66. 您是否有时候能从广播或电视中收到个别交流信息？ _____
如果回答"是"，跳到问题68。如果回答"没有"，继续。

67. 从上帝或者魔鬼那里呢？ _____
如果回答"没有"，跳到问题83。如果回答"有"，继续。

68. 您听到了些什么？ _____

69. 这些声音是否和我的声音一样清晰响亮？ _____

70. 您听到这些声音、噪声、信息等的频率如何？ _____

71. 这些声音出现在1天中的特定时段还是整天都有？ _____
如果只听见噪声，跳到问题80。如果听见说话声音，继续。

72. 您能不能辨别出这些是谁的声音？ _____

73. 声音说什么？ _____

74. 声音是好的还是坏的？ _____

75. 是令人愉快的还是令人不快的？ _____

76. 声音是否干扰了您的思想或活动？ _____

77. 他们有时给您命令或指示吗？ _____
如果回答"不"，跳到问题80。如果回答"是"，继续。

78. 请举个例子。 _____

79. 您一般来说是否遵从这些命令（指示）？ _____

80. 您如何解释这些声音（或噪声）；它们实际上是从哪里来的？ _____

81. 为什么您会有这些体验？ _____

82. 这些体验是正常的吗？ _____

83. 您是否发现有时候普通的东西看起来变得奇特或扭曲？ _____

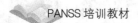
84. Do you sometimes have "visions" or see things that others can't see? _____

IF NO, skip to question 88. IF YES, continue.

85. For example? _____

86. Do these visions seem very real or life-like? _____

87. How often do you have these experiences? _____

88. Do you sometimes smell things that are unusual or that others don't smell? __

IF NO, skip to question 90. IF YES, continue.

89. Please explain. _____

90. Do you get any strange or unusual sensations from your body? _____

IF NO, skip to question 92. IF YES, continue.

91. Tell me about this. _____

Data on "Somatic Concern" (G1)

92. How have you been feeling in terms of your health? _____

IF OTHER THAN "GOOD," skip to question 94. IF "GOOD," continue.

93. Do you consider yourself to be in top health? _____

IF YES, skip to question 95. IF NO, continue.

94. What has been troubling you? _____

95. Do you have any medical illness or disease? _____

96. Has any part of your body been troubling you? _____

IF YES, skip to question 98. IF NO, continue.

97. How is your head? Your heart? Stomach? The rest of your body? _____

98. Could you explain? _____

99. Has your head or body changed in shape or size? _____

IF NO, skip to question 102. IF YES, continue.

100. Please explain. _____

101. What is causing these changes? _____

Data on "Depression" (G6)

102. How has your mood been in the past week: mostly good, mostly bad? _____

IF "MOSTLY BAD," skip to question 104. IF "MOSTLY GOOD," continue.

103. Have there been times in the past week when you were feeling sad or unhappy? _____

IF NO, skip to question 114. IF YES, continue.

104. Is there something in particular that is making you sad? _____

105. How often do you feel sad? _____

84. 您是否有时具有他人没有的"视觉"或看到他人看不到的东西？ _____

如果回答"不"，跳到问题88。如果回答"是"，继续。

85. 请举例。 _____

86. 这些视觉是否看起来非常真实或者生动？ _____

87. 这些体验出现的频率如何？ _____

88. 您是否有时能够闻到一些不寻常的或者是他人闻不到的气味？ _____

如果回答"不"，跳到问题90。如果回答"是"，继续。

89. 请解释。 _____

90. 您是否有来自您身体的奇怪的或者是不寻常的感觉？ _____

如果回答"不"，跳到问题92。如果回答"是"，继续。

91. 跟我讲讲这种感觉。 _____

关于"关注身体健康"(G1)的资料

92. 您感到您的健康情况如何？ _____

如果不是回答"好"，跳到问题94。如果回答"好"，继续。

93. 您是否认为您的健康正处于最好状态？ _____

如果回答"是"，跳到问题95。如果回答"不是"，继续。

94. 是什么正在烦扰您？ _____

95. 您患有任何躯体疾病吗？ _____

96. 您身体的某个部位是否正烦扰着您？ _____

如果回答"是"，跳到问题98。如果回答"不是"，继续。

97. 您的头部如何？您的心脏呢？胃呢？身体的其他部位呢？ _____

98. 您能够解释吗？ _____

99. 您的头部或躯体是否发生了外形或大小的改变？ _____

如果回答"否"，跳到问题102。如果回答"是"，继续。

100. 请解释。 _____

101. 是什么导致了这些变化？ _____

关于"抑郁"(G6)的资料

102. 您过去1周的心情如何：大部分时间好，或大部分时间不好？ _____

如果回答"大部分时间不好"，跳到问题104。如果回答"大部分时间好"，继续。

103. 过去1周中您是否曾经感到忧伤或不愉快？ _____

如果回答"不"，跳到问题114。如果回答"是"，继续。

104. 有什么特殊的事情使您忧伤？ _____

105. 您感到悲伤的频率如何？ _____

106. Just how sad have you been feeling? _____

107. Have you been crying lately? _____

108. Has your mood in any way affected your sleep? _____

109. Has it affected your appetite? _____

110. Do you participate less in activities on account of your mood? _____

111. Have you had any thoughts of harming yourself? _____

IF NO, skip to question 114. IF YES, continue.

112. Any thoughts about ending your life? _____

IF NO, skip to question 114. IF YES, continue.

113. Have you attempted suicide? _____

Data on "Guilt Feelings" (G3) and "Grandiosity" (P5)

114. If you were to compare yourself to the average person, how would you come out: a little better, maybe a little worse, or about the same? _____

IF "BETTER," skip to question 117.

IF "ABOUT THE SAME," skip to question 118.

IF "WORSE," continue.

115. Worse in what ways? _____

116. Just how do you feel about yourself? _____

Skip to question 120.

117. Better in what ways? _____

Skip to question 120.

118. Are you special in some ways? _____

IF NO, skip to question 120. IF YES, continue.

119. In what ways? _____

120. Would you consider yourself gifted? _____

121. Do you have talents or abilities that most people don't have? _____

F NO, skip to question 123. IF YES, continue.

122. Please explain. _____

123. Do you have any special powers? _____

IF NO, skip to question 126. IF YES, continue.

124. What are these? _____

125. Where do these powers come from? _____

126. Do you have extrasensory perception (ESP), or can you read other people's minds? _____

127. Are you very wealthy? _____

IF NO, skip to question 129. IF YES, continue.

106. 您有多悲伤？ _____

107. 您最近有没有哭过？ _____

108. 您的心情是否以某种形式影响了您的睡眠？ _____

109. 它影响了您的食欲吗？ _____

110. 您的心情是否导致您参加的活动减少了？ _____

111. 您是否有任何伤害自己的想法？ _____

如果回答"没有"，跳到问题 114。如果回答"有"，继续。

112. 有没有任何想结束自己生命的想法？ _____

如果回答"没有"，跳到问题 114。如果回答"有"，继续。

113. 您是否曾经尝试过自杀？ _____

关于"自罪感"(G3)和"夸大"(P5)的资料

114. 如果您将自己和一般人进行比较，您的结论如何：好一些，可能差一些，或是差不多？ _____

如果回答"好一些"，跳到问题 117。

如果回答"差不多"，跳到问题 118。

如果回答"差一些"，继续。

115. 在哪些方面差一些？ _____

116. 您对自己的感觉如何？ _____

跳到问题 120。

117. 在哪些方面好一些？ _____

跳到问题 120。

118. 您是否在某些方面很特别？ _____

如果回答"否"，跳到问题 120。如果回答"是"，继续。

119. 在哪些方面？ _____

120. 您认为您自己具有天赋吗？ _____

121. 您是否具有大多数人没有的天资或能力？ _____

如果回答"不"，跳到问题 123。如果回答"是"，继续。

122. 请解释。 _____

123. 您是否具有特殊的力量？ _____

如果回答"否"，跳到问题 126。如果回答"是"，继续。

124. 它们是什么？ _____

125. 这些力量是从哪里来的？ _____

126. 您是否具有超感官知觉(ESP)，或者您能读懂别人的心思吗？ _____

127. 您是否非常富有？ _____

如果回答"否"，跳到问题 129。如果回答"是"，继续。

128. Please explain. _____

129. Can you be considered to be very bright? _____

IF NO, skip to question 131. IF YES, continue.

130. Why would you say so? _____

131. Would you describe yourself as famous? _____

132. Would some people recognize you from TV, radio, or the newspaper? _____

IF NO, skip to question 134. IF YES, continue.

133. Can you tell me about it? _____

134. Are you a religious person? _____

IF NO, skip to question 140. IF YES, continue.

135. Are you close to God? _____

IF NO, skip to question 140. IF YES, continue.

136. Did God assign you some special role or purpose? _____

137. Can you be one of God's messengers or angels? _____

IF NO, skip to question 139. IF YES, continue.

138. What special powers do you have as God's messenger (angel)? _____

139. Do you perhaps consider yourself to be God? _____

140. Do you have some special mission in life? _____

IF NO, skip to question 143. IF YES, continue.

141. What is your mission? _____

142. Who assigned you to that mission? _____

143. Did you ever do something wrong—something you feel bad or guilty about?

_____

IF NO, skip to question 149. IF YES, continue.

144. Just how much does that bother you now? _____

145. Do you feel that you deserve punishment for that? _____

IF NO, skip to question 149. IF YES, continue.

146. What kind of punishment would you deserve? _____

147. Have you at times thought of punishing yourself? _____

IF NO, skip to question 149. IF YES, continue.

148. Have you ever acted on those thoughts of punishing yourself? _____

Data on "Disorientation" (G10)

149. Can you tell me today's date (i. e., the day, month, and year)? _____

IF YES, skip to question 151. IF NO, continue.

150. Can you tell me what day of the week it is? _____

151. What is the name of the place that you are in now? _____

128. 请解释。_____

129. 别人是否认为您名声显赫？_____

如果回答"否"，跳到问题 131。如果回答"是"，继续。

130. 您为什么这么说？_____

131. 您会认为自己很著名吗？_____

132. 有人会从电视、广播或报纸认出您来吗？_____

如果回答"不"，跳到问题 134。如果回答"有"，继续。

133. 您能给我讲讲这方面的事吗？_____

134. 您是教徒吗？_____

如果回答"不是"，跳到问题 140。如果回答"是"，继续。

135. 您是否离上帝（或菩萨）很近？_____

如果回答"不"，跳到问题 140。如果回答"是"，继续。

136. 上帝（或菩萨）是否给您指派了特殊的任务或目的？_____

137. 您是否可能是上帝（或菩萨）的使者或天使之一？_____

如果回答"不"，跳到问题 139。如果回答"是"，继续。

138. 您作为上帝（或菩萨）的使者（天使）具有什么特殊的力量？____

139. 也许您认为自己就是上帝（或菩萨）？_____

140. 您的生命中是否有什么特殊的使命？_____

如果回答"没有"，跳到问题 143。如果回答"有"，继续。

141. 什么是您的使命？_____

142. 是谁给了您这个使命？_____

143. 您曾经做过什么错事——某些令您觉得不好或感到内疚的事情？____

如果回答"没有"，跳到问题 149。如果回答"有"，继续。

144. 现在这些事情烦扰您的程度如何？_____

145. 您是否认为您应该为这些事情接受惩罚？_____

如果回答"不"，跳到问题 149。如果回答"是"，继续。

146. 您应该接受什么样的惩罚？_____

147. 您是否常常出现惩罚自己的想法？_____

如果回答"没有"，跳到问题 149。如果回答"有"，继续。

148. 您是否曾经按照那些惩罚自己的想法采取行动？_____

关于"定向障碍"（G10）的资料

149. 您能告诉我今天的日期（即年、月、日）吗？_____

如果回答"能"，跳到问题 151。如果回答"不能"，继续。

150. 您能告诉我今天是星期几吗？_____

151. 您现在所在的地方叫什么名称？_____

IF NOT HOSPITALIZED, skip to question 154. **IF HOSPITALIZED**, continue.

152. What ward are you on? _____

153. What is the address of where you're now staying? _____

IF ABLE TO TELL, skip to question 155. **IF NOT ABLE TO TELL**, continue.

154. Can you tell me your home address? _____

IF NOT HOSPITALIZED, skip to question 156. **IF HOSPITALIZED**, continue.

155. If someone had to reach you by phone, what number would that person call?

_____

156. If someone had to reach you at home, what number would that person call?

_____

157. What is the name of the doctor who is treating you? _____

IF NOT HOSPITALIZED, skip to question 159. **IF HOSPITALIZED**, continue.

158. Can you tell me who else is on the staff and what they do? _____

159. Do you know who is currently the president (prime minister, etc.)? _____

160. Who is our governor (premier, etc.)? _____

161. Who is the mayor (town supervisor, etc.) of this city (town, etc.)? _____

Data on "Difficulty in Abstract Thinking" (N5)

I'm going to now say a pair of words, and I'd like you to tell me in what important way they're alike. Let's start, for example, with the words "apple" and "banana." How are they alike—what do they have in commen? **IF THE RESPONSE IS THAT "THEY'RE BOTH FRUIT", THEN SAY**: Good. Now what about ...? (*Select three other items from the Similarities list at varying levels of difficulty from Appendix A.*)

IF AN ANSWER IS GIVEN THAT IS CONCRETE, TANGENTIAL, OR IDIOSYNCRATIC (E. G., **"THEY BOTH HAVE SKINS," "YOU CAN EAT THEM," "THEY' RE SMALL," OR "MONKEYS LIKE THEM"), THEN SAY**: OK, but they're both fruit. Now how about ... and ...: how are these alike? (*Select three other items from the Similarities list at varying levels of difficulty from Appendix A.*)

APPENDIX A

Items for Similarities in the evaluation of "Difficulty in Abstract Thinking"

Circle the Similarities Used

1. How are a ball and an orange alike?

2. Apple and banana?

3. Pencil and pen?

4. Nickel and dime?

......

如果未住院,跳到问题 154。如果住院,继续。

152. 您住在什么病房？ _____

153. 您现在所在地方的地址是什么？ _____

如果讲得出,跳到问题 155。如果讲不出,继续。

154. 您能告诉我您的家庭住址吗？ _____

如果未住院,跳到问题 156。如果住院,继续。

155. 假如有人要打电话找您,那么他应该打什么号码？ _____

156. 假如有人要在您家中找您,那么他应该打什么号码？ _____

157. 给您治疗的医生叫什么名字？ _____

如果未住院,跳到问题 159。如果住院,继续。

158. 您还能告诉我哪个工作人员的名字以及他们做什么工作？ _____

159. 您知道现任的国家主席（总统、首相等）是谁吗？ _____

160. 谁是我们的政府领导人（总理等）？ _____

161. 谁是本市的市长（或本镇的镇长等）？ _____

关于"抽象思维困难"(N5)的资料

下面我要说出一对词,请您告诉我它们有什么主要的共同点。现在开始,例如,"苹果"和"香蕉",它们有什么相似处——它们有什么共同的地方？ **如果回答是"它们都是水果",然后你说：很好,那么……和……呢？**（*从附录 A 相似性列表中另选 3 组难度不同的条目。*）

　　如果给出的回答是具体化的、离题的或特质性的（如"它们都有皮","你可以吃","它们是小的",或"猴子喜欢它们"）,然后你说：好的,但是它们都是水果。现在请告诉我……和……,它们有何共同点？（*从附录 A 相似性列表中另选 3 组难度不同的条目。*）

附录 A

评估"抽象思维困难"的相似性条目

圈出使用的相似之处：

1. 皮球和橘子有何相似处？

2. 苹果和香蕉呢？

3. 铅笔和钢笔呢？

4. 分和角呢？

　　……

Note on Appendix A: Similarities are generally assessed by sampling four items at different levels of difficulty (i. e., one item selected from each quarter of the full set). When using the PANSS longitudinally, items should be systematically altered with successive interviews so as to provide different selections from the various levels of difficulty and thus minimize repetition.

Circle the Similarities Used

5. Table and chair?

6. Tiger and elephant?

7. Hat and shirt?

8. Bus and train?

......

9. Arm and leg?

10. Rose and tulip?

11. Uncle and cousin?

12. The sun and the moon?

......

13. Painting and poem?

14. Hilltop and valley?

15. Air and water?

16. Peace and prosperity?

Notes on Similarities responses:

_____

_____

_____

_____

You've probably heard the expression, "Carrying a chip on the shoulder." What does that really mean? There's a very old saying, "Don't judge a book by its cover." What is the deeper meaning of this proverb? (*Select two other proverbs from the list at varying levels of difficulty in Appendix B.*)

APPENDIX B

Items for assessing PROVERB INTERPRETATION in
the evaluation of "Difficulty in Abstract Thinking"

What does the saying mean:

Circle the Similarities Used

1. "Plain as the nose on your face"

附录 A 注释：相似性一般选取 4 个不同难度的条目进行评估（即共有 4 组，每组选 1 个条目）。当纵向使用 PANSS 时，条目应当随着连续的检查而有规则地变换，这样便于提供多种难度水平的不同选择，从而减少重复。

圈出使用的相似之处：

5. 桌子和椅子呢？

6. 老虎和大象呢？

7. 帽子和衬衫呢？

8. 汽车和火车呢？

……

9. 手臂和大腿呢？

10. 玫瑰和郁金香呢？

11. 叔叔和堂兄呢？

12. 太阳和月亮呢？

……

13. 油画和诗歌呢？

14. 山峰和山谷呢？

15. 空气和水呢？

16. 和平和繁荣呢？

相似性回答的记录：

_____

_____

_____

_____

您很可能听说过谚语"开门见山"，它的真正含义是什么？有一句老话叫"黄鼠狼给鸡拜年"，这句谚语的深层含义是什么？（从附录 B 的不同难度组中另选 2 条谚语。）

附录 B

评估"抽象思维困难"中谚语解释的条目

以下说法的含义是什么：

圈出使用的相似之处：

1. "开门见山"

2. "Carrying a chip on your shoulder"

3. "Two heads are better than one"

4. "Too many cooks spoil the broth"

......

5. "Don't judge a book by its cover"

6. "One man's food is another man's poison"

7. "All that glitters is not gold"

Note on Appendix B: Proverb interpretation is generally assessed by sampling four items at different levels of difficulty (i. e., one item selected from each quarter of the full set). When using the PANSS longitudinally, items should be systematically altered with successive interviews so as to provide different selections from the various levels of difficulty and thus minimize repetition.

Circle the Similarities Used

8. "Don't cross the bridge until you come to it"

......

9. "What's good for the goose is good for the gander"

10. "The grass always looks greener on the other side"

11. "Don't keep all your eggs in one basket"

12. "One swallow does not make a summer"

......

13. "A stitch in time saves nine"

14. "A rolling stone gathers no moss"

15. "The acorn never falls far from the tree"

16. "People who live in glass houses should not throw stones at others"

Notes on Proverb responses:

_____

_____

_____

_____

Data on "Lack of Judgment and Insight" (G12)

162. How long have you been in the hospital (clinic, etc.)? _____

163. Why did you come to the hospital (clinic, etc.)? _____

164. Did you need to be in a hospital (clinic, etc.)? _____

IF YES, skip to question 167. IF NO, continue.

165. Did you have a problem that needed treatment? _____

IF NO, skip to question 169. IF YES, continue.

166. Would you say that you had a psychiatric or mental problem? _____

IF NO, skip to question 169. IF YES, continue.

2. "画龙点睛"

3. "泥菩萨过江"

4. "青出于蓝而胜于蓝"

……

5. "种瓜得瓜,种豆得豆"

6. "黄鼠狼给鸡拜年"

7. "猫哭老鼠"

附录 B 注释:谚语解释一般选取 4 个不同难度的条目进行评估(即共有 4 组,每组选1 个条目)。当纵向使用 PANSS 时,条目应当随着连续的检查而有规则地变换,这样便于提供多种难度水平的不同选择,从而减少重复。

圈出使用的相似之处:

8. "对牛弹琴"

……

9. "此地无银三百两"

10. "摸石子过河"

11. "挂羊头卖狗肉"

12. "一箭双雕"

……

13. "磨刀不误砍柴工"

14. "路遥知马力"

15. "亡羊补牢"

16. "画蛇添足"

谚语回答的记录:

_____

_____

_____

_____

关于"判断和自知力缺乏"(G12)的资料

162. 您在这里住院(看门诊等)多久了?　_____

163. 您为何来住院(看门诊等)?　_____

164. 您需要住院(看门诊等)吗?　_____

如果回答"是",跳到问题 167。如果回答"否",继续。

165. 您有什么问题需要治疗吗?　_____

如果回答"没有",跳到问题 169。如果回答"有",继续。

166. 您会说您有精神病或精神方面的问题吗?　_____

如果回答"否",跳到问题 169。如果回答"是",继续。

167. Why? . . . would you say that you had a psychiatric or mental problem? _____

IF NO, skip to question 169. IF YES, continue.

168. Can you tell me about it and what it consisted of? _____

169. In your own opinion, do you need to be taking medicine? _____

IF YES, skip to question 171.

IF NO and unmedicated, skip to question 172.

IF NO and medicated, continue.

170. Why then are you taking medicines? _____

Skip to question 172.

171. Why? . . . Does the medicine help you in any way? _____

172. Do you at this time have any psychiatric or mental problems? _____

IF YES, skip to question 174. IF NO, continue.

173. For what reason are you at the hospital (clinic, etc.)? _____

Skip to question 175.

174. Please explain. _____

175. Just how serious are these problems? _____

IF UNHOSPITALIZED, skip to question 178.

IF HOSPITALIZED, continue.

176. Are you ready yet for discharge from the hospital? _____

177. Do you think you'll be taking medicine for your problems after discharge?

_____

178. What are your future plans? _____

179. What about your longer-range goals? _____

Well, that's about all I have to ask of you now. Are there any questions that you might like to ask of me? Thank you for your cooperation.

167. 为什么？……您说您有精神病或精神方面的问题？ _____

如果回答"否"，跳到问题 169。如果回答"是"，继续。

168. 能否告诉我这方面的情况以及有哪些问题？ _____

169. 依您的意见，您是否需要服药？ _____

如果回答"是"，跳到问题 171。

如果回答"不"，而且未服药，跳到问题 172。

如果回答"不"，但是在服药，继续。

170. 那您为什么服药？ _____

跳到问题 172。

171. 为什么？……药物在某些方面对您有帮助吗？ _____

172. 此刻您是否有精神病或精神方面的问题？ _____

如果回答"是"，跳到问题 174。如果回答"不"，继续。

173. 那您为什么原因而住院（看门诊等）？ _____

跳到问题 175。

174. 请解释。 _____

175. 这些问题有多严重？ _____

如果没有住院，跳到问题 178。

如果住院，继续。

176. 您准备好出院了吗？ _____

177. 您认为出院以后您会继续服药治疗您的问题吗？ _____

178. 您对将来的打算是什么？ _____

179. 您较长远一点的目标呢？ _____

好了，现在我的问题都问完了，您有没有什么问题想问我的？谢谢您的合作。

IQ-PANSS

Informant Questionnaire for the Positive and
Negative Syndrome Scale (IQ-PANSS)

Patient's Name: _____ Patient #: _____

Behavioral Observation Dates: From: ____/____/____ To: ____/____/____

                            mm   dd   yyyy   mm   dd   yyyy

Informant: _____ PANSS Rater: _____

Current medication (s) and dose (s): _____

DIRECTIONS

Please indicate, by putting a checkmark in the space provided, the patient's behavior for the following PANSS items. *Limit your observations* to the patient's behaviors that have been evident during the week immediately preceding the PANSS interview (unless another period of time has been specified). Please pay particular attention to words and/or phrases that appear in boldface print. Please specify observed behaviors for each symptom that is rated as being present. As an example, if a patient has been delusional during the past week or other specified period, list the patient's specific delusion. If he or she has exhibited several delusions, list each one. You may document these behaviors at the bottom of each item in the space provided. Should you require additional space for comments, they may be written on the last page of this booklet. Be sure to indicate the PANSS item to which you are referring by number (e. g. , P1, N5, G3).

In choosing the option that most closely reflects the patient's behavior during this past week (unless another period of time has been specified), please note that choosing **"Questionable pathology"** means that, while the symptom was present (i. e. , the symptom definition applies), it was not present to the degree that any of the other statements could be checked "Yes. "

第四章

IQ-PANSS

阳性和阴性症状量表的知情者调查问卷

患者姓名：＿＿＿＿＿ 患者编号：＿＿＿＿＿

行为观察日期： 从：＿＿月＿＿日＿＿年 至：＿＿月＿＿日＿＿年

知情者：＿＿＿＿＿ PANSS 评定者：＿＿＿＿＿

目前用药和剂量：＿＿＿＿＿＿＿＿＿＿＿＿＿＿＿＿＿＿＿＿＿＿＿

说明

说明与以下 PANSS 条目相对应的患者的行为，请在所提供的空白处打勾。***将您的观察限制*** 在 PANSS 访谈之前一周内（除非已规定另外的时间段）患者的表现行为。请特别注意黑体的单词和（或）词组。请就评定为存在的各项症状列出观察到的行为。例如，如果患者在过去的 1 周或其他指定时间内曾有的妄想症状，请列出患者的具体妄想症状。如果他（或她）表现出多种妄想症状，请列出每一种症状。您可在每个条目下方提供的空白处记录这些行为。如果您的评述需要额外的空白处，可写在本手册的最后一页。请务必按照编号（例如 P1、N5、G3）来说明您所指的 PANSS 条目。

在选择最能反映患者过去 1 周（除非已规定另外的时间段）内的行为的选项时，请注意，选择"**症状可疑**"即意味着，虽然该症状存在（即症状定义适用），但没有达到任何其他陈述均可选择"是"的程度。

TO THE PANSS RATER

The IQ-PANSS has been designed to streamline the process by which informant information is obtained. Please be aware that only those 14 PANSS items that require informant information are included in the IQ-PANSS.

While two PANSS items, Passive/apathetic social withdrawal (N4) and Active social avoidance (G16), are scored exclusively based on information obtained from staff members and/or significant others, informantion reported on the other items included within the IQ-PANSS is to be used in conjunction with data obtained during the Structured Clinical Interview for the PANSS (SCI-PANSS) in arriving at your PANSS ratings. You should contact the IQ-PANSS informant whenever further elaboration and/or clarification of any information is necessary.

P1 DELUSIONS

BELIEFS WHICH ARE UNFOUNDED, UNREALISTIC, AND IDIOSYNCRATIC

1. Symptom is absent _____

2. Questionable pathology; may be at the upper extreme of normal limits _____

3. Are there one or two vague, uncrystallized delusions that are not tenaciously held?
Yes _____   No _____

Do delusions interfere with thinking, social relations, or behavior?

4. Is there an array of poorly formed, unstable delusions or a few well-formed delusions that *occasionally* interfere with thinking, social relations, or behavior?
Yes _____   No _____

5. Are there *numerous* well-formed delusions that *occasionally* interfere with thinking, social relations, or behavior?
Yes _____   No _____

6. Is there a *stable* set of delusions that are crystallized, possibly systematized, tenaciously held, and clearly interfere with thinking, social relations, and behavior?
Yes _____   No _____

7. Is there a stable set of delusions that are *either* highly systematized or very numerous and that *dominate* major facets of the patient's life? If so, do these delusions *frequently* result in inappropriate and irresponsible action, which may jeopardize the safety of the patient or others?
Yes _____   No _____

Observed behaviors:

_____

_____

_____

_____

_____

致 PANSS 评定者

IQ-PANSS 旨在简化据以获得知情者信息的流程。请注意 IQ-PANSS 只包括需要知情者信息的 14 个 PANSS 条目。

虽然被动、淡漠、社交退缩(N4)和主动回避社交(G16)这两项 PANSS 项目是专门根据员工和(或)其他重要人士提供的信息评分,但对 IQ-PANSS 内其他条目的报告信息将与阳性和阴性症状量表的定式化临床检查(SCI-PANSS)期间获得的数据一起使用,以得出您的 PANSS 评分。无论何时需要进一步详尽阐述和(或)澄清任何信息,您都应联系 IQ-PANSS 知情者。

P1 妄想

妄想是指无事实根据、与现实不符、特异的信念。

1. 症状不存在_____

2. 症状可疑,可能是正常范围的上限_____

3. 是否存在一个或两个模糊的、不具体的、并非顽固坚持的妄想?

是_____　　否_____

妄想妨碍患者的思考、社交关系或行为吗?

4. 是否存在一个未完全成形的、不稳定的妄想组合,或几个完全成形的妄想,偶尔妨碍患者的思考、社交关系或行为?

是_____　　否_____

5. 是否有许多完全成形的妄想,偶尔妨碍患者的思考、社交关系或行为?

是_____　　否_____

6. 是否有一整套稳定的、具体的妄想,可能系统化,顽固坚持,且明显妨碍患者的思考、社交关系和行为?

是_____　　否_____

7. 是否有一整套高度系统化或数量众多的稳定的妄想,并支配患者生活的主要方面?如果是,这些妄想是否**经常**会引起患者不恰当的和不负责任的行为,可能因此危及患者或他人的安全?

是_____　　否_____

观察到的行为:

_____

_____

_____

_____

_____

P3 HALLUCINATORY BEHAVIOR

VERBAL REPORT OR BEHAVIOR INDICATING PERCEPTIONS THAT ARE NOT GENERATED BY EXTERNAL STIMULI. THEY MAY BE AUDITORY, VISIUAL, OLFACTORY, OR SOMATIC

1. Symptom is absent _____

2. Questionable pathology; may be at the upper extreme of normal limits _____

3. Are there one or two clearly formed but *infrequent* hallucinations or a number of vague abnormal perceptions that *have not* resulted in distortions of thinking or behavior?

Yes _____   No _____

4. Have hallucinations occurred frequently *but not* continuously with the patient's thinking and behavior being affected only to *a minor* extent?

Yes _____   No _____

5. Have hallucinations occurred frequently and distorted thinking and/or distorted behavior?

Yes _____   No _____

Have hallucinations occurred in more than one sensory modality?

Yes _____   No _____

Has the patient exhibited delusional interpretation of his/her hallucinatory experiences and responded to them emotionally (e. g. , laughter, anger) and, on occasion, verbally as well?

Yes _____   No _____

6. Have hallucinations occurred almost continuously, causing a major disruption of the patient's thinking and behavior?

Yes _____   No _____

Does the patient treat these hallucinations as real perceptions with his/her functioning being impeded by frequent emotional and verbal responses to them?

Yes _____   No _____

7. Has the patient been almost totally preoccupied by hallucinations that virtually dominate thinking and behavior?

Yes _____   No _____

Does the patient have a rigid delusional interpretation of this/these hallucination (s) that provokes verbal and behavioral responses, including obedience to command hallucinations?

Yes _____   No _____

Observed behaviors:

_____

_____

_____

_____

P3　幻觉性行为

幻觉性行为是指患者的语言表达或行为表明存在非外部刺激引起的知觉,这些知觉可能为听觉、视觉、嗅觉或躯体感觉。

1. 症状不存在＿＿＿＿＿

2. 症状可疑,可能是正常范围的上限＿＿＿＿＿

3. 是否有一种或两种清晰但不经常出现的幻觉,或若干模糊异常的知觉,尚未引起患者的思维或行为的失常?

是＿＿＿＿＿否＿＿＿＿＿

4. 幻觉发生是否频繁,但并不持续出现,患者的思维和行为仅受到轻微影响?

是＿＿＿＿＿否＿＿＿＿＿

5. 幻觉是否频繁出现,并致患者的思维和(或)行为的失常?

是＿＿＿＿＿否＿＿＿＿＿

幻觉是否以一种以上感觉形态出现?

是＿＿＿＿＿否＿＿＿＿＿

患者是否对其幻觉体验给予妄想性的解释,并出现情绪反应(例如大笑、发怒),且偶尔出现语言反应?

是＿＿＿＿＿否＿＿＿＿＿

6. 幻觉是否几乎持续发生,以致严重损害患者的思维和行为?

是＿＿＿＿＿否＿＿＿＿＿

患者是否对这些幻觉信以为真,频繁的情绪和语言反应导致其功能障碍?

是＿＿＿＿＿否＿＿＿＿＿

7. 实质上支配患者的思维和行为的幻觉,是否几乎完全占据其思想?

是＿＿＿＿＿否＿＿＿＿＿

患者是否对这个(或这些)幻觉赋予固定的妄想性解释,并引起言语和行为上的反应,包括对命令性幻听的服从?

是＿＿＿＿＿否＿＿＿＿＿

观察到的行为:

＿＿

＿＿

＿＿

＿＿

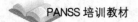

P4   EXCITEMENT

HYPERACTIVITY AS REFLECTED IN ACCELERATED MOTOR BEHAVIOR, HEIGHTENED RESPONSIVITY TO STIMULI, HYPERVIGILANCE, OR EXCESSIVE MOOD LABILITY

1. Symptom is absent _____

2. Questionable pathology; may be at the upper extreme of normal limits _____

3. Has the patient's speech been slightly pressured?

Yes _____   No _____

4. Has the patient exhibited episodic outbursts?

Yes _____   No _____

5. Have you observed significant hyperactivity or frequent outbursts of motor activity by the patient?

Yes _____   No _____

Is it difficult for the patient to sit still for longer than several minutes at a time?

Yes _____   No _____

6. Does marked excitement limit the patient's attention and affect personal functions such as eating and sleeping?

Yes _____   No _____

7. Does marked excitement seriously interfere with eating and sleeping and make interpersonal interactions virtually impossible?

Yes _____   No _____

Does accelerated speech and motor activity result in incoherence and exhaustion?

Yes _____   No _____

Observed behaviors:

_____

_____

_____

_____

_____

P5   GRANDIOSITY

EXAGGERATED SELF-OPINION AND UNREALISTIC CONVICTIONS OF SUPERIORITY, INCLUDING DELUSIONS OF EXTRAORDINARY ABILITIES, WEALTH, KNOWLEDGE, FAME, POWER, AND MORAL RIGHTEOUSNESS

1. Symptom is absent _____

2. Questionable pathology; may be at the upper extreme of normal limits _____

3. Some expansiveness or boastfulness has been evident, but without clear-cut grandiose delusions.

P4　兴奋

活动过度,表现在患者的动作行为加速,对刺激的反应增强,高度警觉或过度的情绪不稳。

1. 症状不存在_____

2. 症状可疑,可能是正常范围的上限_____

3. 患者言谈是否一直有轻微的紧迫感?

是_____否_____

4. 患者是否一直表现出短暂的爆发?

是_____否_____

5. 您是否观察到患者有明显的活动过度或频繁的动作行为爆发?

是_____否_____

患者是否很难一次保持坐姿超过数分钟?

是_____否_____

6. 明显的兴奋是否阻碍患者的注意力并影响个人功能诸如饮食和睡眠?

是_____否_____

7. 明显的兴奋是否严重妨碍饮食和睡眠,并使得人际交往实际上变得不可能?

是_____否_____

言语和动作行为的加速是否导致语无伦次和精疲力竭?

是_____否_____

观察到的行为:

_____

_____

_____

_____

P5　夸大

夸张己见及不现实的优势观念,包括一些妄想,如非凡的能力、财富、知识、名望、权力和道德正义。

1. 症状不存在_____

2. 症状可疑,可能是正常范围的上限_____

3. 患者有一些明显的自大或自夸,但没有明确的夸大妄想。

Yes _____ No _____

4. The patient feels distinctly and unrealistically superior to others.

Yes _____ No _____

Does the patient possess some poorly formed delusions about special status or abilities?

Yes _____ No _____

Has the patient acted on these delusions?

Yes _____ No _____

5. Has the patient expressed clear-cut delusions concerning remarkable abilities, status, or power that have influenced attitude but not behavior?

Yes _____ No _____

6. Has the patient expressed clear-cut delusions of remarkable superiority that involve more than one parameter such as wealth, knowledge, fame, etc.?

Yes _____ No _____

Have these delusions notably affected the patient's interactions and/or been acted upon?

Yes _____ No _____

7. Have the patient's thinking, interactions, and behavior been dominated by multiple delusions of amazing ability, wealth, knowledge, fame, power, and/or moral stature?

Yes _____ No _____

If so, has this taken on a bizarre quality?

Yes _____ No _____

Observed behaviors (if applicable, list grandiose delusions):

_____

_____

_____

_____

_____

P6 SUSPICIOUSNESS/PERSECUTION

UNREALISTIC OR EXAGGERATED IDEAS OF PERSECUTION, AS REFLECTED IN GUARDEDNESS, A DISTRUSTFUL ATTITUDE, SUSPICIOUS HYPERVIGILANCE, OR FRANK DELUSIONS THAT OTHERS MEAN ONE HARM

1. Symptom is absent _____

2. Questionable pathology; may be at the upper extreme of normal limits _____

3. Does the patient present with a guarded or even openly distrustful attitude?

Yes _____ No _____

If so, would you say that the patient's thoughts, interactions, and behavior are only minimally affected by this attitude?

是_____否_____

4. 患者明确地和不切实际地感到自己比他人优越。

是_____否_____

患者是否有一些尚未成形的关于特殊地位或能力的妄想?

是_____否_____

患者依照这些妄想行事吗?

是_____否_____

5. 患者是否表达出有明确的关于非凡能力、地位或权利的妄想,这些妄想已影响其态度,但不影响其行为?

是_____否_____

6. 患者是否表达出有明确的显著优势妄想,涉及一个以上的项目,例如财富、知识、名望等?

是_____否_____

这些妄想是否显著影响患者的人际交往,和(或)患者是否根据这些妄想行事?

是_____否_____

7. 患者的思维、人际交往和行为是否已受多重妄想的支配,这些妄想包括惊人的能力、财富、知识、名望、权力和(或)道德高度?

是_____否_____

如果是,是否具有古怪的性质?

是_____否_____

观察到患者的行为(如适用列出的夸大妄想):

_____

_____

_____

_____

_____

P6 猜疑或被害感

猜疑或被害感是指患者具有不现实或夸大的被害观念,表现在防卫、不信任态度、多疑的高度戒备或是认为他人对其有伤害的非常明显的妄想。

1. 症状不存在_____

2. 症状可疑,可能是正常范围的上限_____

3. 患者是否表现出防卫或甚至公开的不信任态度?

是_____否_____

如果是,您是否认为这种态度对患者的思维、交往和行为只产生最小限度的影响?

Yes _____   No _____

4. Has the patient's distrustfulness been clearly evident and intruded on his/her behavior?

Yes _____   No _____

Has there been evidence of persecutory delusions?

Yes _____   No _____

Has there been evidence of loosely formed persecutory delusions that have not affected the patient's attitude or interpersonal relations?

Yes _____   No _____

5. Has the patient showed marked distrustfulness that has led to *major* disruptions of interpersonal relations?

Yes _____   No _____

Have there been clear-cut persecutory delusions that have limited impact on interpersonal relations and behavior?

Yes _____   No _____

6. Has the patient exhibited clear-cut pervasive delusions of persecution that may be systematized and significantly interfere with interpersonal relations?

Yes _____   No _____

7. Have you noticed a network of systematized persecutory delusions that dominate the patient's thinking, social relations, and behavior?

Yes _____   No _____

Observed behaviors (if applicable, list persecutory delusions):

_____

_____

_____

_____

_____

P7 HOSTILITY

VERBAL AND NONVERBAL EXPRESSIONS OF ANGER AND RESENTMENT, INCLUDING SARCASM, PASSIVE-AGGRESSIVE BEHAVIOR, VERBAL ABUSE, AND ASSAULTIVENESS

1. Symptom is absent _____

2. Questionable pathology; may be at the upper extreme of normal limits _____

3. Does the patient communicate indirect or restrained anger (e. g., sarcasm, disrespect, hostile expressions, and occasional irritability)?

Yes _____   No _____

4. Does the patient present with an overtly hostile attitude, showing frequent

是_____ 否_____

4. 患者的不信任感是否很明显并且妨碍他(或她)的行为?

是_____ 否_____

是否有被害妄想的证据?

是_____ 否_____

是否存在结构松散的被害妄想,但尚未影响患者的态度或人际关系?

是_____ 否_____

5. 患者是否表现出明显的不信任感,已致人际关系造成严重破坏?

是_____ 否_____

是否有明确的被害妄想,已对人际关系和行为造成一定程度的影响?

是_____ 否_____

6. 患者是否表现出明确的泛化的被害妄想,可能是系统化的且显著地妨碍人际关系?

是_____ 否_____

7. 您是否注意到有一整套系统性被害妄想支配患者的思维、社交关系和行为?

是_____ 否_____

观察到的行为(如适用,列出被害妄想):

_____

_____

_____

_____

P7 敌对性

敌对性是指患者以愤怒和怨恨的言语和非言语表达,包括讥讽、被动攻击行为、辱骂和袭击。

1. 症状不存在_____

2. 症状可疑,可能是正常范围的上限_____

3. 患者是否间接地或经过克制地表示愤怒(如讥讽、不尊敬、表达敌意及偶尔易激惹)?

是_____ 否_____

4. 患者是否存在明显的敌对态度,经常表现易激惹及直接表达愤怒或怨恨?

irritability and directly expressing anger or resentment?

Yes _____ No _____

5. Has the patient been highly irritable and occasionally verbally abusive or threatening?

Yes _____ No _____

6. Has uncooperativeness and verbal abuse or threats seriously impacted on the patient's social relations?

Yes _____ No _____

Has the patient been violent and destructive without having been physically assaultive toward others?

Yes _____ No _____

7. Has marked anger resulted in extreme uncooperativeness that has either precluded other interactions or led to episode (s) of physical assault toward others?

Yes _____ No _____

Observed behaviors:

_____

_____

_____

_____

N2 EMOTIONAL WITHDRAWAL

LACK OF INTEREST IN, INVOLVEMENT WITH, AND AFFECTIVE COMMITMENT TO LIFE'S EVENTS

1. Symptom is absent _____

2. Questionable pathology; may be at the upper extreme of normal limits _____

3. Does the patient usually lack initiative?

Yes _____ No _____

Does the patient show deficient interest in surrounding events?

Yes _____ No _____

4. Is the patient generally distanced emotionally from the milieu and its challenges?

Yes _____ No _____

Can the patient be engaged in interactions when encouraged?

Yes _____ No _____

5. Is the patient clearly detached emotionally from persons and events in the milieu, resisting all efforts at engagement?

Yes _____ No _____

是_____否_____

5. 患者是否高度易激惹,而且偶尔有辱骂或言语威胁?

是_____否_____

6. 不合作和辱骂或言语威胁是否已严重影响患者的社交关系?

是_____否_____

患者是否具有暴力和破坏性行为,但没有对他人进行人身攻击?

是_____否_____

7. 明显的愤怒是否已造成极度不合作,以致拒绝与他人交往或对他人进行人身攻击?

是_____否_____

观察到的行为:

_____

_____

_____

_____

N2 情绪退缩

情绪退缩是指患者对生活事件缺乏兴趣、参与和情感投入。

1. 症状不存在_____

2. 症状可疑,可能是正常范围的上限_____

3. 患者是否经常缺乏主动性?

是_____否_____

患者是否显得对周围事件缺乏兴趣?

是_____否_____

4. 患者是否总体上对周围环境及环境变化有情感隔阂?

是_____否_____

患者受鼓励后能否参与交往?

是_____否_____

5. 患者是否对周围的人和事有明显的情感疏远,抵制所有的参与努力?

是_____否_____

Is it the case that the patient appears distant, docile, and purposeless but can, nevertheless, be involved in communication at least briefly?

Yes _____ No _____

Does the patient tend to personal needs, even if he/she sometimes needs assistance?

Yes _____ No _____

6. Have you noticed a marked deficiency of interest and emotional commitment that has resulted in limited conversation with others and frequent neglect of personal functions, for which the patient requires supervision?

Yes _____ No _____

7. Has the patient been almost totally withdrawn, uncommunicative, and neglectful of personal needs, resulting from a profound lack of interest and emotional commitment?

Yes _____ No _____

Observed behaviors:

_____

_____

_____

_____

_____

N4   PASSIVE/APATHETIC SOCIAL WITHDRAWAL

DIMINISHED INTEREST AND INITIATIVE IN SOCIAL INTERACTIONS DUE TO PASSIVITY, APATHY, ANERGY, OR AVOLITION. THIS LEADS TO REDUCED INTERPERSONAL INVOLVEMENTS AND NEGLECT OF ACTIVITIES OF DAILY LIVING

1. Symptom is absent _____

2. Questionable pathology; may be at the upper extreme of normal limits _____

3. Does the patient show occasional interest in social activities but poor initiative? For example, does the patient usually engage with others only when approached first by them?

Yes _____ No _____

4. Does the patient passively go along with most social activities but in a disinterested or mechanical way, tending to recede into the background?

Yes _____ No _____

5. Does the patient passively participate in only a minority of activities and show virtually no interest or initiative?

Yes _____ No _____

Does the patient generally spend little time with others?

Yes _____ No _____

6. Does the patient tend to be apathetic and isolated, participating very rarely in

患者是否显得疏远、温顺和漫无目的,但不管怎样却至少可进行短暂的交流?

是_____ 否_____

患者是否倾向于个人需求,即使有时需要帮助?

是_____ 否_____

6. 您是否注意到患者有明显的缺乏兴趣和情感投入,导致与他人交谈有限,并且经常忽略个人功能,因此患者需要监督?

是_____ 否_____

7. 患者是否因兴趣和情感投入的极度缺乏导致其几乎完全退缩,无法与他人交谈,并忽略个人需求?

是_____ 否_____

观察到的行为:

_____

_____

_____

_____

_____

N4　被动性或淡漠性社交退缩

因被动、淡漠、缺乏精力或意志力使患者对社会交往的兴趣和主动性下降,这导致人际投入的减少及对日常活动的忽视。

1. 症状不存在_____

2. 症状可疑,可能是正常范围的上限_____

3. 患者是否显示对社交活动偶有兴趣,但主动性较差? 例如,通常只有在他人先主动表示时才会参与?

是_____ 否_____

4. 患者是否被动地参与大部分的社交活动,但以无兴趣或机械的方式出现,倾向于退缩到不显眼的地方?

是_____ 否_____

5. 患者是否仅被动参与少数活动,且实际上显得毫无兴趣或主动性?

是_____ 否_____

患者通常只花很少时间与他人相处吗?

是_____ 否_____

6. 患者是否趋于淡漠和孤立,极少参与社交活动?

social activities?

Yes _____ No _____

Is he/she occasionally neglectful of personal needs?

Yes _____ No _____

Does the patient have very few spontaneous social contacts?

Yes _____ No _____

7. Has the patient been profoundly apathetic, socially isolated, and personally neglectful. (e.g., very poor Activities of Daily Living-such as making bed, brushing teeth, bathing)?

Yes _____ No _____

Observed behaviors:

_____

_____

_____

_____

* **Note: This is one of two PANSS items that are scored exclusively based on information obtained from staff members and/or significant others, so the level of severity chosen here will be used as the PANSS rating for this item.**

G5 MANNERISMS AND POSTURING

UNNATURAL MOVEMENTS OR POSTURE AS CHARACTERIZED BY AN AWKWARD, STILTED, DISORGANIZED, OR BIZARRE APPEARANCE

1. Symptom is absent _____

2. Questionable pathology; may be at the upper extreme of normal limits _____

3. Has the patient's movements been slightly awkward or have you noticed a minor rigidity of posture?

Yes _____ No _____

4. Have you noticed that the patient's movements are *notably* awkward or disjointed or that the patient has maintained an unnatural posture for brief periods?

Yes _____ No _____

5. Has the patient engaged in *occasional* bizarre motoric rituals?

Yes _____ No _____

Have you noticed the patient engaging in a contorted posture or, perhaps, an abnormal position that has been sustained for extended periods?

Yes _____ No _____

6. Has the patient engaged in frequent repetition of bizarre rituals, mannerisms, or stereotyped movements or, perhaps, has sustained a contorted posture for extended period?

Yes _____ No _____

是_____否_____

他(她)是否偶尔忽视个人需求?

是_____否_____

患者是否很少有自发的社交接触?

是_____否_____

7. 患者是否一直以极度的淡漠状态,与世隔绝,且忽视个人需求(例如,铺床、刷牙、洗澡等日常生活行为习惯极差)?

是_____否_____

观察到的行为:

_____

_____

_____

_____

_____

*注:这是两个 PANSS 项目之一,专门根据员工和(或)其他重要人士提供的信息评分,因此此处所选的严重程度将作为该项目的 PANSS 评分使用。

G5　装相和作态

装相和作态是指患者所表现为不自然的动作或姿势,以笨拙、做作、紊乱或古怪表现为特征。

1. 症状不存在_____

2. 症状可疑,可能是正常范围的上限_____

3. 患者的动作是否有点笨拙或您是否注意到其姿势有些僵硬?

是_____否_____

4. 您是否注意到患者的动作明显笨拙或不连贯,或患者短时间保持一种不自然的姿势?

是_____否_____

5. 患者偶有古怪的仪式性动作吗?

是_____否_____

您是否注意到患者摆出扭曲的姿势,或可能长时间保持一种异常的姿势?

是_____否_____

6. 患者是否经常重复出现古怪的仪式性动作、装相或刻板动作,或可能长时间保持一种扭曲的姿势?

是_____否_____

7. Has the patient's functioning been seriously impaired by virtually constant involvement in ritualistic, manneristic, or stereotyped movements or by an unnatural fixed posture that is sustained most of the time?

Yes _____   No _____

Observed behaviors:

_____

_____

_____

_____

_____

G6 DEPRESSION

FEELINGS OF SADNESS, DISCOURAGEMENT, HELPLESSNESS, AND PESSIMISM

1. Symptom is absent _____

2. Questionable pathology; may be at the upper extreme of normal limits _____

3. Has the patient expressed some sadness or discouragement only upon questioning and without any evidence of depression in general attitude or demeanor?

Yes _____   No _____

4. Has there been any evidence of distinct feelings of sadness or hopelessness, that may have been spontaneously divulged?

Yes _____   No _____

If so, is it the case that this depressed mood *has not* had a major impact on behavior or social functioning, and the patient can usually be cheered up?

Yes _____   No _____

5. Is the patient's depressed mood associated with obvious sadness, pessimism, loss of social interest, psychomotor retardation, and has it interfered somewhat in appetite and sleep?

Yes _____   No _____

6. Has the patient's markedly depressed mood been associated with sustained feelings of misery, *occasional* crying, hopelessness, and worthlessnes?

Yes _____   No _____

Has it significantly interfered with appetite and/or sleep as well as in normal motor and social functions, with possible signs of self-neglect being evident?

Yes _____   No _____

7. Have the patient's depressive feelings *seriously* interfered with most major functions? Manifestations include frequent crying, pronounced somatic symptoms, impaired concentration, psychomotor retardation, social disinterest, self-neglect, possible depressive and/or nihilistic delusions, and/or possible suicidal thoughts or actions?

Yes _____   No _____

7. 患者的功能是否因几乎持续不断的仪式性动作、装相或刻板动作,或大部分时间保持一种不自然的固定姿势,而严重受损?

是_____否_____

观察到的行为:

_____

_____

_____

_____

_____

G6　抑郁

抑郁是指患者表现为悲伤、沮丧、无助和悲观厌世的感觉。

1. 症状不存在_____

2. 症状可疑,可能是正常范围的上限_____

3. 患者是否只在被问及时才表示出有些悲伤或沮丧,但总的态度或行为举止没有抑郁表现?

是_____否_____

4. 是否有明显感到患者有悲伤或绝望的迹象,而这可能是自然流露出来的?

是_____否_____

若是,这种抑郁心境是否尚未对患者的行为或社会功能造成重大影响,而且患者通常还能高兴起来?

是_____否_____

5. 患者的抑郁心境是否伴有明显的悲伤、悲观厌世、失去社交兴趣和精神运动迟滞,而且是否对食欲和睡眠有些妨碍?

是_____否_____

6. 患者明显的抑郁心境是否已伴有持续的痛苦感、偶尔哭泣、绝望和无价值感?

是_____否_____

该情绪是否已严重妨碍食欲和(或)睡眠以及正常运动和社会功能,可能伴有明显的自我忽视的迹象?

是_____否_____

7. 患者的抑郁感觉是否已严重妨碍大部分主要功能? 表现包括经常哭泣,明显的躯体症状,注意力损害,精神运动迟滞,失去社交兴趣,自我忽视,可能有抑郁和(或)虚无妄想,和(或)可能有自杀意念或行为?

是_____否_____

Observed behaviors:

_____

_____

_____

_____

G7   MOTOR RETARDATION

REDUCTION IN MOTOR ACTIVITY AS REFLECTED IN SLOWING OR LESSENING OF MOVEMENTS AND SPEECH, DIMINISHED RESPONSIVENESS TO STIMULI, AND REDUCED BODY TONE

1. Symptom is absent _____

2. Questionable pathology; may be at the upper extreme of normal limits _____

3. Has there been a slight but noticeable diminution in the patient's rate of movements and speech (e. g., the patient may be somewhat underproductive in conversation and gestures)?

Yes _____   No _____

4. Has the patient been *clearly slow* in movements?

Yes _____   No _____

Has the patient's speech been characterized by poor productivity, including long response latency, extended pauses, or slow pace?

Yes _____   No _____

5. Have you noticed a *marked* reduction in motor activity that has rendered communication highly unproductive or, perhaps, has delimited functioning in social and occupational situations?

Yes _____   No _____

Is it the case that the patient could usually be found sitting or lying down?

Yes _____   No _____

6. Have the patient's movements been extremely slow, resulting in a minimum of activity and speech with the patient spending his/her day essentially sitting idly or lying down?

Yes _____   No _____

7. Is it the case that the patient has been almost completely immobile and virtually unresponsive to external stimuli?

Yes _____   No _____

Observed behaviors:

_____

_____

_____

_____

_____

观察到的行为：

_____

_____

_____

_____

G7　运动迟缓

运动迟缓是指患者运动活动减少,表现在动作和言语的减慢或减少,对刺激的反应减弱及体质变弱。

1. 症状不存在_____

2. 症状可疑,可能是正常范围的上限_____

3. 患者的动作和讲话速度是否轻微但明显减慢(例如,患者的谈话内容和姿势可能有点不足)?

是_____否_____

4. 患者的动作是否明显减慢?

是_____否_____

患者的讲话特点是否为讲话内容不足,包括反应期延长、停顿延长或语速缓慢?

是_____否_____

5. 您是否注意到患者运动活动显著减少,已导致交谈内容非常不足,或已影响到社交和职业功能?

是_____否_____

患者是否常被发现发呆着或躺着?

是_____否_____

6. 患者的动作是否极其缓慢,导致极少活动和讲话,患者基本上整天呆坐或躺着?

是_____否_____

7. 患者是否几乎完全不动,并且对外界刺激毫无反应?

是_____否_____

观察到的行为：

_____

_____

_____

_____

_____

G8 UNCOOPERATIVENESS

ACTIVE REFUSAL TO COMPLY WITH THE WILL OF SIGNIFICANT OTHERS, INCLUDING THE INTERVIEWER, HOSPITAL STAFF, OR FAMILY, WHICH MAY BE ASSOCIATED WITH DISTRUST, DEFENSIVENESS, STUBBORNNESS, NEGATIVISM, REJECTOIN OF AUTHORITY, HOSTILITY, OR BELLIGERENCE

1. Symptom is absent _____

2. Questionable pathology; may be at the upper extreme of normal limits _____

3. The patient complies with an attitude of resentment, impatience, or sarcasm.

Yes _____   No _____

4. The patient occasionally refuses outright to comply with normal social demands, such as making his/her bed, attending scheduled programs, etc.

Yes _____   No _____

Does the patient project a hostile, defensive, or negative attitude?

Yes _____   No _____

Can the patient usually be worked with?

Yes _____   No _____

5. Has the patient been frequently noncompliant with the demands of his/her milieu?

Yes _____   No _____

Is the patient characterized by others as an "outcast" or as having "a serious attitude problem"?

Yes _____   No _____

6. Has the patient been highly uncooperative, negativistic, or possibly belligerent?

Yes _____   No _____

Has the patient refused to comply with most social demands?

Yes _____   No _____

7. Has the patient's active resistance *seriously* impacted on virtually all major areas of functioning? For example, the patient may refuse to join in any social activities, tend to personal hygiene, converse with family or staff or participate even briefly in an interview?

Yes _____   No _____

Observed behaviors:

_____

_____

_____

_____

_____

G8　不合作

患者主动拒绝顺从其他重要人物的意愿,包括检查者、医务人员或家属,可能伴有不信任、防御、固执、消极、抵制权威、敌对或好斗。

1. 症状不存在_____

2. 症状可疑,可能是正常范围的上限_____

3. 患者以一种愤恨、不耐烦或讥讽的态度服从。

是_____否_____

4. 患者偶尔直率地拒绝服从正常的社会要求,如整理自己的床铺、参加安排好的活动等。

是_____否_____

患者是否表现出敌对、防御或否定的态度?

是_____否_____

患者在通常情况下是否可以共事?

是_____否_____

5. 患者是否经常不遵从周围环境的要求?

是_____否_____

患者是否被他人描述为"被遗弃者"或有"严重的态度问题"?

是_____否_____

6. 患者是否高度不合作、否定,或可能好斗?

是_____否_____

患者是否拒绝服从大部分社会要求?

是_____否_____

7. 患者的主动抵制是否严重影响患者参与几乎所有主要的功能领域? 例如,患者可能拒绝参加任何社交活动,不注意个人卫生,不与家属或工作人员谈话,或甚至拒绝参与简短的会谈?

是_____否_____

观察到的行为:

_____

_____

_____

_____

_____

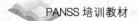

G14 POOR IMPULSE CONTROL

DISORDERED REGULATION AND CONTROL OF ACTION ON INNER URGES, RESULTING IN SUDDEN, UNMODULATED, ARBITRARY, OR MISDIRECTED DISCHARGE OF TENSION AND EMOTIONS WITHOUT CONCERN ABOUT CONSEQUENCES

1. Symptom is absent _____

2. Questionable pathology; may be at the upper extreme of normal limits _____

3. The patient has tended to be easily angered and frustrated when facing stress or denied gratification but rarely acts on impulse.

Yes _____ No _____

4. Has the patient been angered and verbally abusive with minimal provocation?

Yes _____ No _____

Has the patient been occasionally threatening or destructive?

Yes _____ No _____

Has the patient been involved in any physical confrontations or minor brawls?

Yes _____ No _____

5. Has the patient exhibited repeated impulsive episodes involving verbal abuse, destruction of property, or physical threats?

Yes _____ No _____

Has the patient had any episodes that have involved serious assault for which the patient has required isolation, physical restraint, or p.r.n. sedation?

Yes _____ No _____

6. Has the patient been frequently impulsively aggressive, threatening, demanding, and destructive, without any apparent consideration of consequences?

Yes _____ No _____

Has the patient exhibited either assaultive or sexually offensive behavior?

Yes _____ No _____

Has the patient behaviorally responded to hallucinatory commands?

Yes _____ No _____

7. Has the patient exhibited homicidal attacks, sexual assaults, repeated brutality, or self-destructive behavior?

Yes _____ No _____

Has the patient required *constant* direct supervision or external constraints because of inability to control dangerous impulses?

Yes _____ No _____

Observed behaviors:

_____

G14 冲动控制障碍

对内在冲动反应的调节和控制障碍,导致不顾后果的、突然的、无法调节的、肆意的或误导的紧张和情绪的宣泄。

1. 症状不存在_____

2. 症状可疑,可能是正常范围的上限_____

3. 在面对应激或不如意时,患者容易出现愤怒和受挫感,但很少冲动行事。

是_____否_____

4. 患者是否对轻微的挑衅就会愤怒和谩骂?

是_____否_____

患者是否偶尔出现威胁性或破坏性行为?

是_____否_____

患者是否发生任何有关的身体冲突或程度较轻的吵架?

是_____否_____

5. 患者是否反复出现冲动,包括谩骂、毁物或肢体威胁?

是_____否_____

患者是否有任何严重攻击行为,以致患者需要隔离、身体约束或必要时给予镇静剂?

是_____否_____

6. 患者是否经常不计后果地出现攻击、威胁、强人所难和破坏性行为?

是_____否_____

患者是否表现出攻击性或性攻击行为?

是_____否_____

患者是否对幻听命令做出行为反应?

是_____否_____

7. 患者是否曾出现致命的攻击、性侵犯、反复的残暴行为或自残行为?

是_____否_____

患者是否因不能控制其危险性冲动而需要不断的直接监管或外部约束?

是_____否_____

观察到的行为:

_____

_____

_____

_____

_____

G16　ACTIVE SOCIAL AVOIDANCE

DIMINISHED SOCIAL INVOLVEMENT ASSOCIATED WITH UNWARRANTED FEAR, HOSTILITY, OR DISTRUST

1. Symptom is absent _____

2. Questionable pathology; may be at the upper extreme of normal limits _____

3. The patient seems ill at ease in the presence of others and prefers to spend time alone, although he/she participates in social functions when required.

Yes _____　No _____

4. Has the patient grudgingly attended all or most social activities?

Yes _____　No _____

Has the patient needed to be persuaded to attend social activities?

Yes _____　No _____

Has the patient terminated his/her participation on account of anxiety, suspiciousness, or hostility?

Yes _____　No _____

5. Is it the case that the patient has either fearfully or angrily kept away from many social interactions, despite the efforts of others to engage him/her?

Yes _____　No _____

Does the patient tend to spend unstructured time alone due to unwarranted fear, hostility, or distrust?

Yes _____　No _____

6. Has the patient participated in very few social activities because of unwarranted fear, hostility, or distrust?

Yes _____　No _____

When approached, has the patient shown a strong tendency to break off interactions and generally isolate him/herself from others?

Yes _____　No _____

7. Is it the case that the patient could not be engaged in social activities because of pronounced fears, hostility, or persecutory delusions and, to the extent possible, has avoided all interactions and remained isolated from others?

Yes _____　No _____

Observed behaviors:

_____

_____

_____

_____

_____

G16　主动回避社交

主动回避社交是指患者由于无根据的恐惧、敌意或不信任而减少社交参与。

1. 症状不存在_____

2. 症状可疑,可能是正常范围的上限_____

3. 患者在别人面前似乎显得不自在,并且喜欢独自消磨时光,尽管他(她)在要求下仍会参加社交活动。

是_____否_____

4. 患者是否非常勉强地参加所有或大部分社交活动?

是_____否_____

患者是否需要经劝说才参加社交活动?

是_____否_____

患者是否因焦虑、猜疑或敌意而中止参与活动?

是_____否_____

5. 尽管他人努力邀请他(或她)参加社交活动,患者是否仍因恐惧或愤怒而远离许多社会交往?

是_____否_____

患者是否因无根据的恐惧、敌意或不信任而倾向于独自消磨空闲时间?

是_____否_____

6. 患者是否因无根据的恐惧、敌意或不信任而极少参加社交活动?

是_____否_____

当他人接近时,患者是否表现出强烈的中止交往的倾向,并且通常离群索居?

是_____否_____

7. 患者是否因极度恐惧、敌意或被害妄想而不参加社交活动,而且尽可能地回避所有的交往并离群索居?

是_____否_____

观察到的行为:

_____

_____

_____

_____

_____

＊ **Note**: **This is one of two PANSS items that are scored exclusively based on information obtained from staff members and/or significant others, so the level of severity chosen here will be used as the PANSS rating for this item.**

NOTES

＊＊BE SURE TO SPECIFY THE ITEM(S) FOR WHICH YOU ARE PROVIDING ADDITIONAL INFORMATION

_____

_____

_____

_____

_____

＊注：这是两个 PANSS 项目之一，专门根据员工和(或)其他重要人士提供的信息评分，因此此处所选的严重程度将作为该项目的 PANSS 评分使用。

注　意

＊＊请务必指明您提供的额外信息是针对哪一项

培训流程

通常,一个完整的 PANSS 培训流程包括以下步骤:

一 —— 培训前准备

(1) 培训材料:含 PANSS 基本资料,培训课件,小测验,访谈模拟案例(书面材料为主),评分模拟案例(录像资料为主),一致性测试用表格,投票器。

(2) 培训老师:资格审查,预演和评估,确定培训时长(通常为 3 小时)。

(3) 培训场地:确定人数和空间,多媒体预演,投票器预演。

(4) 培训对象:基本信息收集(姓名、身份证号码、医师资格证和执业证、单位、是否参加过 PANSS 培训等),资格审查(精神科实际工作时间),建立/更新评分员数据库。

(5) 考试材料:访谈考试案例(含脚本制作和评估,标准化受试者的培训和评估),访谈考核表设计和确认,访谈考核通过标准的确定,评分考试案例(含脚本和录像的制作,各条目标准分的讨论和确认),评分考核通过标准的确认。

二 —— 培训现场

(1) 量表简介。

(2) 各条目介绍和小测验。

(3) 访谈培训:模拟案例,角色扮演。通常 3 人一组,评分员、受试者和督导者角色轮换。

(4) 评分培训:模拟案例,各条目逐一分析和讨论。

(5) 提问与答疑。

(6) 访谈考试:标准化受试者对评分员的评分,通过者方可进行评分考试。

(7) 评分考试:录像 1,一致性测试;不通过者录像 2,再次进行一致性测试。

三 —— 培训完成后

(1) 评分员证书:通过访谈考试＋评分考试者取得评分员证书,通常有效期为一年。

(2) 更新评分员数据库,建立评分质控计划,通常 2 月一次。

(3) 持续培训:一年期满,需再次培训(可根据质控情况减免部分或全部培训内容),

更新评分员证书。

（4）准备后续培训。

说明：PANSS 量表培训包括两个部分：访谈培训和评分培训，尤其需要强调访谈的重要性，因为依据合格的访谈才能获取完整、可靠的相关信息，这是准确评分的基础。因此，从事精神科实际工作时间不足两年的医生不适合成为评分员。

通过访谈和评分考试的评分员，在实际临床研究工作中，是否依然能够正确使用 PANSS，需要实施质控评估。应当收集评分员的实际工作量，例如，一个评分员在一年内仅对 1 名受试者进行了 3 次 PANSS 评分，就很有必要再次接受培训；可采用各种质控方法，常用的质控评估有两类：一、经患者知情同意后录音、录像，或远程同步语音或视频会议；二、对评分员已完成的量表评分进行数据分析和模型拟合。如果质控评估发现存在频繁而且严重的评分错误，可暂停评分员资格，要求其进行再次培训；而对于评分质量较好的评分员，持续培训时，可以视情况减免部分或全部培训内容。

对于评分质量要求高的临床研究，例如关键性研究（pivotal study），可以采用中心化量表评估的手段。

一个评分员获得评分员证书后，在一年有效期内参与多个研究，无须再次培训。

参考文献

［1］ Stephen R. Marder, John M. Davis, Guy Chouinard. The Effects of Risperidone on the Five Dimensions of Schizophrenia Derived by Factor Analysis: Combined Results of the North American Trials ［J］. J Clin Psychiatiry. 1997;58(12): 538 - 546.

［2］ www. cnki. com. cn/CJFD/CJFD_index. htm.

［3］ Kay SR, Opler LA, Fiszbein A. *Positive and Negative Syndrome Scale（PANSS）Manual*［M］. North Tonawanda, NY: Multi-Health Systems Inc; 1999.

［4］ 何燕玲,诸索宇,张明园译. 阳性与阴性症状量表(中文版)手册(内部出版物)［M］.

［5］ Stanley RK, Lewis AO. Structured clinical interview for th positive and negative syndrome scale (SCI-PANSS)［M］. 1988.

［6］ Lewis A O, Paul M R. Informant questionnaire for the positive and negative syndrome scale (IQ-PANSS)［M］.（Copyright © 1999. Muti-Health Systems Inc.）.

PANSS 一致性测试用表格

录像编号 _____

P1.妄想	1	2	3	4	5	6	7
P2.概念紊乱(联想散漫)	1	2	3	4	5	6	7
P3.幻觉行为	1	2	3	4	5	6	7
P4.兴奋	1	2	3	4	5	6	7
P5.夸大	1	2	3	4	5	6	7
P6.猜疑/迫害	1	2	3	4	5	6	7
P7.敌意	1	2	3	4	5	6	7
N1.情感迟钝	1	2	3	4	5	6	7
N2.情绪退缩	1	2	3	4	5	6	7
N3.(情感)交流障碍	1	2	3	4	5	6	7
N4.被动/淡漠的社交退缩	1	2	3	4	5	6	7
N5.抽象思维困难	1	2	3	4	5	6	7
N6.交流缺乏自发性和流畅性	1	2	3	4	5	6	7
N7.刻板思考	1	2	3	4	5	6	7
G1.关注身体健康	1	2	3	4	5	6	7
G2.焦虑	1	2	3	4	5	6	7
G3.自罪感	1	2	3	4	5	6	7
G4.身体紧张	1	2	3	4	5	6	7
G5.装相和作态	1	2	3	4	5	6	7
G6.抑郁	1	2	3	4	5	6	7
G7.动作迟滞	1	2	3	4	5	6	7
G8.不合作	1	2	3	4	5	6	7
G9.不寻常思维内容	1	2	3	4	5	6	7
G10.定向障碍	1	2	3	4	5	6	7
G11.注意障碍	1	2	3	4	5	6	7
G12.判断和自制力缺乏	1	2	3	4	5	6	7
G13.意志障碍	1	2	3	4	5	6	7
G14.冲动控制障碍	1	2	3	4	5	6	7
G15.先占观念	1	2	3	4	5	6	7
G16.主动回避社交	1	2	3	4	5	6	7

总分 □□□

单位/中心号 _____

姓名 _____ 日期 _____

PANSS 一致性测试用表格

录像编号 _____

P1. 妄想	1	2	3	4	5	6	7
P2. 概念紊乱(联想散漫)	1	2	3	4	5	6	7
P3. 幻觉行为	1	2	3	4	5	6	7
P4. 兴奋	1	2	3	4	5	6	7
P5. 夸大	1	2	3	4	5	6	7
P6. 猜疑/迫害	1	2	3	4	5	6	7
P7. 敌意	1	2	3	4	5	6	7
N1. 情感迟钝	1	2	3	4	5	6	7
N2. 情绪退缩	1	2	3	4	5	6	7
N3. (情感)交流障碍	1	2	3	4	5	6	7
N4. 被动/淡漠的社交退缩	1	2	3	4	5	6	7
N5. 抽象思维困难	1	2	3	4	5	6	7
N6. 交流缺乏自发性和流畅性	1	2	3	4	5	6	7
N7. 刻板思考	1	2	3	4	5	6	7
G1. 关注身体健康	1	2	3	4	5	6	7
G2. 焦虑	1	2	3	4	5	6	7
G3. 自罪感	1	2	3	4	5	6	7
G4. 身体紧张	1	2	3	4	5	6	7
G5. 装相和作态	1	2	3	4	5	6	7
G6. 抑郁	1	2	3	4	5	6	7
G7. 动作迟滞	1	2	3	4	5	6	7
G8. 不合作	1	2	3	4	5	6	7
G9. 不寻常思维内容	1	2	3	4	5	6	7
G10. 定向障碍	1	2	3	4	5	6	7
G11. 注意障碍	1	2	3	4	5	6	7
G12. 判断和自制力缺乏	1	2	3	4	5	6	7
G13. 意志障碍	1	2	3	4	5	6	7
G14. 冲动控制障碍	1	2	3	4	5	6	7
G15. 先占观念	1	2	3	4	5	6	7
G16. 主动回避社交	1	2	3	4	5	6	7

总分　□□□

单位/中心号_____

姓名_____　　　日期_____

PANSS 一致性测试用表格

录像编号_____

P1.妄想	1	2	3	4	5	6	7
P2.概念紊乱（联想散漫）	1	2	3	4	5	6	7
P3.幻觉行为	1	2	3	4	5	6	7
P4.兴奋	1	2	3	4	5	6	7
P5.夸大	1	2	3	4	5	6	7
P6.猜疑/迫害	1	2	3	4	5	6	7
P7.敌意	1	2	3	4	5	6	7
N1.情感迟钝	1	2	3	4	5	6	7
N2.情绪退缩	1	2	3	4	5	6	7
N3.(情感)交流障碍	1	2	3	4	5	6	7
N4.被动/淡漠的社交退缩	1	2	3	4	5	6	7
N5.抽象思维困难	1	2	3	4	5	6	7
N6.交流缺乏自发性和流畅性	1	2	3	4	5	6	7
N7.刻板思考	1	2	3	4	5	6	7
G1.关注身体健康	1	2	3	4	5	6	7
G2.焦虑	1	2	3	4	5	6	7
G3.自罪感	1	2	3	4	5	6	7
G4.身体紧张	1	2	3	4	5	6	7
G5.装相和作态	1	2	3	4	5	6	7
G6.抑郁	1	2	3	4	5	6	7
G7.动作迟滞	1	2	3	4	5	6	7
G8.不合作	1	2	3	4	5	6	7
G9.不寻常思维内容	1	2	3	4	5	6	7
G10.定向障碍	1	2	3	4	5	6	7
G11.注意障碍	1	2	3	4	5	6	7
G12.判断和自制力缺乏	1	2	3	4	5	6	7
G13.意志障碍	1	2	3	4	5	6	7
G14.冲动控制障碍	1	2	3	4	5	6	7
G15.先占观念	1	2	3	4	5	6	7
G16.主动回避社交	1	2	3	4	5	6	7

总分 □□□

单位/中心号_____

姓名_____ 日期_____

PANSS 一致性测试用表格

录像编号_____

P1.妄想	1	2	3	4	5	6	7
P2.概念紊乱(联想散漫)	1	2	3	4	5	6	7
P3.幻觉行为	1	2	3	4	5	6	7
P4.兴奋	1	2	3	4	5	6	7
P5.夸大	1	2	3	4	5	6	7
P6.猜疑/迫害	1	2	3	4	5	6	7
P7.敌意	1	2	3	4	5	6	7
N1.情感迟钝	1	2	3	4	5	6	7
N2.情绪退缩	1	2	3	4	5	6	7
N3.(情感)交流障碍	1	2	3	4	5	6	7
N4.被动/淡漠的社交退缩	1	2	3	4	5	6	7
N5.抽象思维困难	1	2	3	4	5	6	7
N6.交流缺乏自发性和流畅性	1	2	3	4	5	6	7
N7.刻板思考	1	2	3	4	5	6	7
G1.关注身体健康	1	2	3	4	5	6	7
G2.焦虑	1	2	3	4	5	6	7
G3.自罪感	1	2	3	4	5	6	7
G4.身体紧张	1	2	3	4	5	6	7
G5.装相和作态	1	2	3	4	5	6	7
G6.抑郁	1	2	3	4	5	6	7
G7.动作迟滞	1	2	3	4	5	6	7
G8.不合作	1	2	3	4	5	6	7
G9.不寻常思维内容	1	2	3	4	5	6	7
G10.定向障碍	1	2	3	4	5	6	7
G11.注意障碍	1	2	3	4	5	6	7
G12.判断和自制力缺乏	1	2	3	4	5	6	7
G13.意志障碍	1	2	3	4	5	6	7
G14.冲动控制障碍	1	2	3	4	5	6	7
G15.先占观念	1	2	3	4	5	6	7
G16.主动回避社交	1	2	3	4	5	6	7

总分　□□□

单位/中心号_____

姓名_____　　　　日期_____

PANSS 一致性测试用表格

录像编号 _____

P1. 妄想	1	2	3	4	5	6	7
P2. 概念紊乱（联想散漫）	1	2	3	4	5	6	7
P3. 幻觉行为	1	2	3	4	5	6	7
P4. 兴奋	1	2	3	4	5	6	7
P5. 夸大	1	2	3	4	5	6	7
P6. 猜疑/迫害	1	2	3	4	5	6	7
P7. 敌意	1	2	3	4	5	6	7
N1. 情感迟钝	1	2	3	4	5	6	7
N2. 情绪退缩	1	2	3	4	5	6	7
N3. （情感）交流障碍	1	2	3	4	5	6	7
N4. 被动/淡漠的社交退缩	1	2	3	4	5	6	7
N5. 抽象思维困难	1	2	3	4	5	6	7
N6. 交流缺乏自发性和流畅性	1	2	3	4	5	6	7
N7. 刻板思考	1	2	3	4	5	6	7
G1. 关注身体健康	1	2	3	4	5	6	7
G2. 焦虑	1	2	3	4	5	6	7
G3. 自罪感	1	2	3	4	5	6	7
G4. 身体紧张	1	2	3	4	5	6	7
G5. 装相和作态	1	2	3	4	5	6	7
G6. 抑郁	1	2	3	4	5	6	7
G7. 动作迟滞	1	2	3	4	5	6	7
G8. 不合作	1	2	3	4	5	6	7
G9. 不寻常思维内容	1	2	3	4	5	6	7
G10. 定向障碍	1	2	3	4	5	6	7
G11. 注意障碍	1	2	3	4	5	6	7
G12. 判断和自制力缺乏	1	2	3	4	5	6	7
G13. 意志障碍	1	2	3	4	5	6	7
G14. 冲动控制障碍	1	2	3	4	5	6	7
G15. 先占观念	1	2	3	4	5	6	7
G16. 主动回避社交	1	2	3	4	5	6	7

总分 □□□

单位/中心号 _____

姓名 _____ 日期 _____

PANSS 一致性测试用表格

录像编号_____

P1. 妄想	1	2	3	4	5	6	7
P2. 概念紊乱(联想散漫)	1	2	3	4	5	6	7
P3. 幻觉行为	1	2	3	4	5	6	7
P4. 兴奋	1	2	3	4	5	6	7
P5. 夸大	1	2	3	4	5	6	7
P6. 猜疑/迫害	1	2	3	4	5	6	7
P7. 敌意	1	2	3	4	5	6	7
N1. 情感迟钝	1	2	3	4	5	6	7
N2. 情绪退缩	1	2	3	4	5	6	7
N3. (情感)交流障碍	1	2	3	4	5	6	7
N4. 被动/淡漠的社交退缩	1	2	3	4	5	6	7
N5. 抽象思维困难	1	2	3	4	5	6	7
N6. 交流缺乏自发性和流畅性	1	2	3	4	5	6	7
N7. 刻板思考	1	2	3	4	5	6	7
G1. 羊注身体健康	1	2	3	4	5	6	7
G2. 焦虑	1	2	3	4	5	6	7
G3. 自罪感	1	2	3	4	5	6	7
G4. 身体紧张	1	2	3	4	5	6	7
G5. 装相和作态	1	2	3	4	5	6	7
G6. 抑郁	1	2	3	4	5	6	7
G7. 动作迟滞	1	2	3	4	5	6	7
G8. 不合作	1	2	3	4	5	6	7
G9. 不寻常思维内容	1	2	3	4	5	6	7
G10. 定向障碍	1	2	3	4	5	6	7
G11. 注意障碍	1	2	3	4	5	6	7
G12. 判断和自制力缺乏	1	2	3	4	5	6	7
G13. 意志障碍	1	2	3	4	5	6	7
G14. 冲动控制障碍	1	2	3	4	5	6	7
G15. 先占观念	1	2	3	4	5	6	7
G16. 主动回避社交	1	2	3	4	5	6	7

总分 □□□

单位/中心号_____

姓名_____   日期_____

PANSS 一致性测试用表格

录像编号＿＿＿＿＿＿＿＿＿＿＿＿＿＿＿＿＿

P1.妄想	1	2	3	4	5	6	7
P2.概念紊乱(联想散漫)	1	2	3	4	5	6	7
P3.幻觉行为	1	2	3	4	5	6	7
P4.兴奋	1	2	3	4	5	6	7
P5.夸大	1	2	3	4	5	6	7
P6.猜疑/迫害	1	2	3	4	5	6	7
P7.敌意	1	2	3	4	5	6	7
N1.情感迟钝	1	2	3	4	5	6	7
N2.情绪退缩	1	2	3	4	5	6	7
N3.(情感)交流障碍	1	2	3	4	5	6	7
N4.被动/淡漠的社交退缩	1	2	3	4	5	6	7
N5.抽象思维困难	1	2	3	4	5	6	7
N6.交流缺乏自发性和流畅性	1	2	3	4	5	6	7
N7.刻板思考	1	2	3	4	5	6	7
G1.关注身体健康	1	2	3	4	5	6	7
G2.焦虑	1	2	3	4	5	6	7
G3.自罪感	1	2	3	4	5	6	7
G4.身体紧张	1	2	3	4	5	6	7
G5.装相和作态	1	2	3	4	5	6	7
G6.抑郁	1	2	3	4	5	6	7
G7.动作迟滞	1	2	3	4	5	6	7
G8.不合作	1	2	3	4	5	6	7
G9.不寻常思维内容	1	2	3	4	5	6	7
G10.定向障碍	1	2	3	4	5	6	7
G11.注意障碍	1	2	3	4	5	6	7
G12.判断和自制力缺乏	1	2	3	4	5	6	7
G13.意志障碍	1	2	3	4	5	6	7
G14.冲动控制障碍	1	2	3	4	5	6	7
G15.先占观念	1	2	3	4	5	6	7
G16.主动回避社交	1	2	3	4	5	6	7

总分　□□□

单位/中心号＿＿＿＿＿＿＿＿＿＿＿＿＿＿＿＿＿

姓名＿＿＿＿＿＿＿＿＿＿＿＿＿＿＿　　　日期＿＿＿＿＿＿＿＿＿＿＿＿＿＿＿

PANSS 一致性测试用表格

录像编号_____

	1	2	3	4	5	6	7
P1. 妄想	1	2	3	4	5	6	7
P2. 概念紊乱（联想散漫）	1	2	3	4	5	6	7
P3. 幻觉行为	1	2	3	4	5	6	7
P4. 兴奋	1	2	3	4	5	6	7
P5. 夸大	1	2	3	4	5	6	7
P6. 猜疑/迫害	1	2	3	4	5	6	7
P7. 敌意	1	2	3	4	5	6	7
N1. 情感迟钝	1	2	3	4	5	6	7
N2. 情绪退缩	1	2	3	4	5	6	7
N3. (情感)交流障碍	1	2	3	4	5	6	7
N4. 被动/淡漠的社交退缩	1	2	3	4	5	6	7
N5. 抽象思维困难	1	2	3	4	5	6	7
N6. 交流缺乏自发性和流畅性	1	2	3	4	5	6	7
N7. 刻板思考	1	2	3	4	5	6	7
G1. 关注身体健康	1	2	3	4	5	6	7
G2. 焦虑	1	2	3	4	5	6	7
G3. 自罪感	1	2	3	4	5	6	7
G4. 身体紧张	1	2	3	4	5	6	7
G5. 装相和作态	1	2	3	4	5	6	7
G6. 抑郁	1	2	3	4	5	6	7
G7. 动作迟滞	1	2	3	4	5	6	7
G8. 不合作	1	2	3	4	5	6	7
G9. 不寻常思维内容	1	2	3	4	5	6	7
G10. 定向障碍	1	2	3	4	5	6	7
G11. 注意障碍	1	2	3	4	5	6	7
G12. 判断和自制力缺乏	1	2	3	4	5	6	7
G13. 意志障碍	1	2	3	4	5	6	7
G14. 冲动控制障碍	1	2	3	4	5	6	7
G15. 先占观念	1	2	3	4	5	6	7
G16. 主动回避社交	1	2	3	4	5	6	7

总分　□□□

单位/中心号_____

姓名_____　　　日期_____

PANSS 一致性测试用表格

录像编号_____

	1	2	3	4	5	6	7
P1. 妄想	1	2	3	4	5	6	7
P2. 概念紊乱(联想散漫)	1	2	3	4	5	6	7
P3. 幻觉行为	1	2	3	4	5	6	7
P4. 兴奋	1	2	3	4	5	6	7
P5. 夸大	1	2	3	4	5	6	7
P6. 猜疑/迫害	1	2	3	4	5	6	7
P7. 敌意	1	2	3	4	5	6	7
N1. 情感迟钝	1	2	3	4	5	6	7
N2. 情绪退缩	1	2	3	4	5	6	7
N3. (情感)交流障碍	1	2	3	4	5	6	7
N4. 被动/淡漠的社交退缩	1	2	3	4	5	6	7
N5. 抽象思维困难	1	2	3	4	5	6	7
N6. 交流缺乏自发性和流畅性	1	2	3	4	5	6	7
N7. 刻板思考	1	2	3	4	5	6	7
G1. 关注身体健康	1	2	3	4	5	6	7
G2. 焦虑	1	2	3	4	5	6	7
G3. 自罪感	1	2	3	4	5	6	7
G4. 身体紧张	1	2	3	4	5	6	7
G5. 装相和作态	1	2	3	4	5	6	7
G6. 抑郁	1	2	3	4	5	6	7
G7. 动作迟滞	1	2	3	4	5	6	7
G8. 不合作	1	2	3	4	5	6	7
G9. 不寻常思维内容	1	2	3	4	5	6	7
G10. 定向障碍	1	2	3	4	5	6	7
G11. 注意障碍	1	2	3	4	5	6	7
G12. 判断和自制力缺乏	1	2	3	4	5	6	7
G13. 意志障碍	1	2	3	4	5	6	7
G14. 冲动控制障碍	1	2	3	4	5	6	7
G15. 先占观念	1	2	3	4	5	6	7
G16. 主动回避社交	1	2	3	4	5	6	7

总分　□□□
单位/中心号_____
姓名_____　　　　日期_____

PANSS 一致性测试用表格

录像编号 _____

P1. 妄想	1	2	3	4	5	6	7
P2. 概念紊乱（联想散漫）	1	2	3	4	5	6	7
P3. 幻觉行为	1	2	3	4	5	6	7
P4. 兴奋	1	2	3	4	5	6	7
P5. 夸大	1	2	3	4	5	6	7
P6. 猜疑/迫害	1	2	3	4	5	6	7
P7. 敌意	1	2	3	4	5	6	7
N1. 情感迟钝	1	2	3	4	5	6	7
N2. 情绪退缩	1	2	3	4	5	6	7
N3. （情感）交流障碍	1	2	3	4	5	6	7
N4. 被动/淡漠的社交退缩	1	2	3	4	5	6	7
N5. 抽象思维困难	1	2	3	4	5	6	7
N6. 交流缺乏自发性和流畅性	1	2	3	4	5	6	7
N7. 刻板思考	1	2	3	4	5	6	7
G1. 关注身体健康	1	2	3	4	5	6	7
G2. 焦虑	1	2	3	4	5	6	7
G3. 自罪感	1	2	3	4	5	6	7
G4. 身体紧张	1	2	3	4	5	6	7
G5. 装相和作态	1	2	3	4	5	6	7
G6. 抑郁	1	2	3	4	5	6	7
G7. 动作迟滞	1	2	3	4	5	6	7
G8. 不合作	1	2	3	4	5	6	7
G9. 不寻常思维内容	1	2	3	4	5	6	7
G10. 定向障碍	1	2	3	4	5	6	7
G11. 注意障碍	1	2	3	4	5	6	7
G12. 判断和自制力缺乏	1	2	3	4	5	6	7
G13. 意志障碍	1	2	3	4	5	6	7
G14. 冲动控制障碍	1	2	3	4	5	6	7
G15. 先占观念	1	2	3	4	5	6	7
G16. 主动回避社交	1	2	3	4	5	6	7

总分 □□□

单位/中心号 _____

姓名 _____   日期 _____

PANSS 一致性测试用表格

录像编号_____

P1.妄想	1	2	3	4	5	6	7
P2.概念紊乱(联想散漫)	1	2	3	4	5	6	7
P3.幻觉行为	1	2	3	4	5	6	7
P4.兴奋	1	2	3	4	5	6	7
P5.夸大	1	2	3	4	5	6	7
P6.猜疑/迫害	1	2	3	4	5	6	7
P7.敌意	1	2	3	4	5	6	7
N1.情感迟钝	1	2	3	4	5	6	7
N2.情绪退缩	1	2	3	4	5	6	7
N3.(情感)交流障碍	1	2	3	4	5	6	7
N4.被动/淡漠的社交退缩	1	2	3	4	5	6	7
N5.抽象思维困难	1	2	3	4	5	6	7
N6.交流缺乏自发性和流畅性	1	2	3	4	5	6	7
N7.刻板思考	1	2	3	4	5	6	7
G1.关注身体健康	1	2	3	4	5	6	7
G2.焦虑	1	2	3	4	5	6	7
G3.自罪感	1	2	3	4	5	6	7
G4.身体紧张	1	2	3	4	5	6	7
G5.装相和作态	1	2	3	4	5	6	7
G6.抑郁	1	2	3	4	5	6	7
G7.动作迟滞	1	2	3	4	5	6	7
G8.不合作	1	2	3	4	5	6	7
G9.不寻常思维内容	1	2	3	4	5	6	7
G10.定向障碍	1	2	3	4	5	6	7
G11.注意障碍	1	2	3	4	5	6	7
G12.判断和自制力缺乏	1	2	3	4	5	6	7
G13.意志障碍	1	2	3	4	5	6	7
G14.冲动控制障碍	1	2	3	4	5	6	7
G15.先占观念	1	2	3	4	5	6	7
G16.主动回避社交	1	2	3	4	5	6	7

总分 □□□

单位/中心号_____

姓名_____ 日期_____

PANSS 一致性测试用表格

录像编号 _____

P1.妄想	1	2	3	4	5	6	7
P2.概念紊乱(联想散漫)	1	2	3	4	5	6	7
P3.幻觉行为	1	2	3	4	5	6	7
P4.兴奋	1	2	3	4	5	6	7
P5.夸大	1	2	3	4	5	6	7
P6.猜疑/迫害	1	2	3	4	5	6	7
P7.敌意	1	2	3	4	5	6	7
N1.情感迟钝	1	2	3	4	5	6	7
N2.情绪退缩	1	2	3	4	5	6	7
N3.(情感)交流障碍	1	2	3	4	5	6	7
N4.被动/淡漠的社交退缩	1	2	3	4	5	6	7
N5.抽象思维困难	1	2	3	4	5	6	7
N6.交流缺乏自发性和流畅性	1	2	3	4	5	6	7
N7.刻板思考	1	2	3	4	5	6	7
G1.关注身体健康	1	2	3	4	5	6	7
G2.焦虑	1	2	3	4	5	6	7
G3.自罪感	1	2	3	4	5	6	7
G4.身体紧张	1	2	3	4	5	6	7
G5.装相和作态	1	2	3	4	5	6	7
G6.抑郁	1	2	3	4	5	6	7
G7.动作迟滞	1	2	3	4	5	6	7
G8.不合作	1	2	3	4	5	6	7
G9.不寻常思维内容	1	2	3	4	5	6	7
G10.定向障碍	1	2	3	4	5	6	7
G11.注意障碍	1	2	3	4	5	6	7
G12.判断和自制力缺乏	1	2	3	4	5	6	7
G13.意志障碍	1	2	3	4	5	6	7
G14.冲动控制障碍	1	2	3	4	5	6	7
G15.先占观念	1	2	3	4	5	6	7
G16.主动回避社交	1	2	3	4	5	6	7

总分　□□□

单位/中心号 _____

姓名 _____　　　　　　日期 _____